LET ME INTRODUCE YOU:

THREESOMES, TALES OF LEVERS, AND MOVEMENT.

JENN PILOTTI
ADARIAN BARR

Printed in the United States.

Cover design by Maddi Jura
Book design by Asya Blue Design
Photographs by Rob Pleas and Emily Aygun

ISBN 979-8-9873395-0-3 Paperback
ISBN 979-8-9873395-1-0 Ebook

TABLE OF CONTENTS

ABOUT US

HOW IT CAME TO BE

Jenn's story:

Once upon a time, more than two decades ago, I began a career in fitness. I quickly realized something was missing, and so I went searching, searching for the magic system to explain why people moved the way they did and how I could help people move in a way that felt more coordinated, athletic, and easier.

I searched the lands (and the Interwebz) far and wide. I spent thousands of dollars learning systems only to become frustrated as I realized the systems weren't answering my questions or explaining what I saw. And so, me being me, I began studying neuroscience, anatomy, physiology, and psychology, determined to find the missing piece, the glue that tied all of these concepts together.

I was pretty sure I had a decent grasp on things until the fateful day I met Adarian Barr. I quickly realized I knew less than I thought and he knew more than I did. This was not only irritating, it was also fascinating—what he was teaching made sense and clearly needed to be distilled into a book (because that seems to my solution to everything—read the book, or write the book).

Here we are, two years after that chance encounter, thousands of words and countless DMs later, with a story about moving; specifically, how it works. In the words of Fred Rogers, "I feel so strongly that deep and simple is far more essential than shallow and complex." The concepts are simple, but profound. They strip away the complexity that the field of human movement and fitness is often fraught with, leaving instead the idea that the production of movement is based on an innate wisdom, an intelligence that doesn't require a lot of interference. This inherent intelligence can not only make the experience of moving feel easier and more powerful, but can create a sense of autonomy and self-agency. It can give the person operating the body a sense of freedom and deep strength.

The following pages are my attempt to give you the tools needed to create a sense of freedom in your body. That freedom is often accompanied by a sense of empowerment and joy as you reclaim the body strength and intelligence you have within you. I hope you enjoy exploring these ideas as much as I enjoyed learning about them, and that they assist you in your path towards finding elation with movement.

Adarian's story:

Introductions are about both new relationships and reviving old ones. The person, or object, you are being introduced to offers opportunities to expand or confirm your experiences.

When introduced to a person that you did not previously know, you are presented with the opportunity to expand your knowledge of the person and see what you wish to make of this new relationship; and, how this new relationship might fit into your experiences.

If reintroduced to a person you previously had a relationship with or knew about, you again get the chance to expand your knowledge and determine what you wish to make of this relationship.

I started the journey of movement discovery back in high school. I was a high-level athlete, and my skill level exceeded that of the coaches' capacity to improve. They actually gave me a book on triple jumps and informed me that I would have to become a student of the sport and myself, if I wanted to improve, as they could do no more. Off I went to the library to find more books on anything that was moving related, from horses to airplanes to sea otters.

I am truly appreciative of what they did. They introduced me to movement exploration, and with that newfound relationship I chose to make it fit my experience of becoming a better athlete.

I have been an athlete for decades. When I was younger and just playing, I had no idea of what an athlete was; I thought some children were just having more fun than others.

I also thought some children just like to play differently, like those that like to roughhouse versus those that chase butterflies. I also thought playing was a way to explore my environment, from walking down steep hills to climbing rocks and trees.

Around the fifth grade I was selected to be on a track team, which is when I started to learn about being an athlete. Once again, I thought it was just play until I lost. I had just been introduced into a new relationship: competition with consequences.

Throughout life you are introduce to foods, sex, anger, trust, and so much more. With each of these introductions comes an experience, and it's your ability to choose what you want to make of this new relationship. You could enjoy the food or sex, or you could not.

Movement is something you're introduced to from day one of conception. You have no choices in what to do with this new relationship. Once born, you can choose to do what you want in this new introduced environment.

Here is to being introduced to me; I trust this new relationship will be a positive one.

CHAPTER 1

FEEL THE SENSATION

You know that moment, just before elation, when you are experiencing a deep connection with your body? You are one with the moment, time stands still, and all you can hear is the percussion that comes with the movement?

Nope, I'm not talking about sex. I am talking about the experience of moving freely, which can certainly happen during sex, but this book isn't about that (it would have been in a different section of the bookstore if it were). This book is about how movement works and how you can move well, with a sense of athleticism, autonomy, and intention.

I know, I know. Why should you read another book that's all about anatomy and biomechanics? What will you get from more boring science terms that are hard to apply while you are running, lifting, dancing, or just flowing?

Because this isn't a book about anatomy and biomechanics.

Sure, there will be the occasional reference to body parts or biomechanics, but this is a book about movement principles; principles that are rooted in the physical sciences and will allow you to not just survive, but thrive in whatever movement setting suits your fancy. We believe that conveying these ideas in a simple way is more beneficial than bogging you down with terms that are hard to remember, and we want you to read this and feel inspired about what you can do. Because you can do so much more than you realize.

How it all came to be:

In June of 2020, in the middle of the pandemic and during the brief moment that residents of the state of California were allowed to function in a semi-normal fashion as long as masks and social distancing were practiced, I hosted a small gathering of movement professionals at my studio in Carmel. It was organized by my friend Chris Ruffolo, a woman so passionate about movement she runs a free website called Thinkmovement when she isn't teaching high school students physical education. She is the PE teacher I wish I had, focusing on interaction and allowing the teenagers who aren't interested in traditional sports to explore movement through game play and improvisation. To say she thinks outside the box would be an understatement—she doesn't see boxes, she sees kaleidoscopes.

When she asked if I was open to people outside of our normal group coming, I said sure, as long as we didn't have more than ten people (2020 will forever be immortalized as the year of small gatherings). I glanced at the final list when she sent it over and noticed I didn't recognize two of the names. I wondered who she'd invited, then moved on without giving it a second thought.

Two weeks later, on a Saturday, I was introduced to Adarian Barr. I was kicking off the morning with an exploration on the connection between the feet and the pelvis (more about that in chapter 3). He was lecturing right after me on arches. I figured he was talking about foot arches, and I assumed there was logic to the schedule so our talks would complement each other in some way.

He concisely and quickly explain the power of the transverse arch (a topic we will explain more fully later), so we struck up conversation, which led to a collaboration. It was during this collaboration that I realized his view of looking at the human body and movement was not only very similar with my philosophies, but was filling in gaps through physics principles that I didn't realize were missing. While I had been exposed to them before, they hadn't been taught in a way that was simple and accessible to the field of movement.

It starts sometime around pressure:

What characterizes a good kiss? If the kiss is light, fleeting, it doesn't feel like much. It's barely detected by the skin or lips and can feel irritating, like a brush of air that didn't quite land.

If it's too hard, it's uncomfortable. It's hard to lean into or reciprocate. But somewhere between these two extremes is that sweet spot, where there is just enough pressure by the other person that you can press back, giving and receiving with the lips in a dance whose music is the application and reception of pressure.

Pressure is the way the brain and the body talk to each other. Pressure is detected by the specialized cells in the muscles, tendons, ligaments, and joints that tell the brain things like how much a joint is bent and how much tension is on a muscle.

The brain takes that information and determines how you move. When someone kisses you too lightly, your brain isn't sure how to interpret the meaning; too forcefully, and the brain detects maybe something is amiss and you shouldn't kiss back. But when the pressure is just right, the brain detects an optimal amount of input and corresponds with just the right output. "The input is the output," Adarian told me when I was pestering him for a more direct definition of how this all works. "It has to come from you."

This means you are the one who generates the internal pressure the brain detects when you are doing an activity like running. This pressure comes from a lot of places, including your respiratory system (a.k.a. how you're breathing), and the internal force you are able to generate. You can think of this as your internal strength. When you run, the result of this internal pressure is everything from what your gait looks like to how fast you move through space. In case you missed it one paragraph ago: the input is the output.

Fortunately, understanding pressure and how to detect pressure is a skill that can be developed, just like dead lifting or running or doing a handstand. It's an internal skill that requires focus, observation, and dropping into your body.

With the ability to detect pressure comes the ability to change pressure. When you begin to tinker with the amount of pressure that is acting upon your structure, how you move changes. You become more aware of how you are moving and what you are moving, which means your body awareness increases. Your timing also changes and timing, along with sequencing and coordination, is a critical piece to an often neglected piece of athleticism: speed.

Moving fast not only enables you to get from point A to point B quickly; it allows you to be agile and powerful. It gives you the ultimate sense of physical control and freedom.

But before we get too far ahead of ourselves, know this: tapping into your inner athlete, the one who can move fast without fear, starts with how well you detect pressure. Are you willing to fine-tune how you kiss, allowing your lips to meet your partner's lips in a way that is pleasurable and reciprocal? These things rarely happen perfectly the first time. They require some work. Detecting your internal pressure is no different. It takes practice, but once you find your internal rhythm, the outcome is immeasurably rewarding.

Defining the term pressure:

I keep using the term pressure, and I gave you a concrete example of the experience of pressure, but what does it actually mean?

Pressure is defined as the amount of force applied over a specific area. This should make sense; when you get a deep tissue massage, the amount of force applied in a specific area, let's say your left-middle back region, is high. Because the pressure is high, it might feel uncomfortable or overwhelming, like you don't know what to do with the force that is being applied directly on your skin.

If, on the other hand, you are getting a gentle spa massage, what one of my massage therapist friends like to call a "fluff and buff," the pressure on your left-middle back would be a lot less. It will feel different because it is different; how you respond to the two experiences will differ.

I know, I know. These ideas seem repetitive. But they are important, so bear with me as we take a little closer look at what, exactly, it means to create internal pressure.

Another way to think about internal pressure is as a form of compression. In your car, compression occurs when the piston travels to compress the fuel mixture. This squeezes the volume of the fuel mixture, which increases pressure, easily allowing the spark to create internal combustion. It all starts with the spark.

When the blood flows:

What happens when you read an erotic poem or watch a suggestive scene in a movie? Blood flow increases to your genitalia, causing swelling. This increased swelling makes the area more sensitive to pressure (Woodard & Diamond, 2009). What happens next involves either: taking advantage of this heightened sensitivity by applying external pressure, or waiting until the pressure dissipates.

Fifty to sixty percent of you is fluid (Brinkman et al., 2022). This fluid is located both in and outside the cells. It controls the body's internal balance; the fluids location depends on pressure inside and outside of the body. Why is it hard to breathe while exercising at high altitude? Because the atmospheric pressure is reduced, which changes the pressure of the air you inhale. Your body responds by circulating more blood throughout your entire system (Grover et al., 1986). Changing pressure one place changes pressure somewhere else. And what does this do? It changes the input, which changes the output.

When you are experiencing something that suits your particular brand of sexual interest, the sensation that comes from pressure or touch is heightened by your increased sensitivity (Paterson et al., 2013). Generally, the outcome is something pleasurable.

This example of pleasure is in direct juxtaposition to what happens when an area is injured. Blood flow still increases because of various pressure changes in the body, causing swelling and inflammation. This allows the circulatory system to deliver oxygen and carry away waste from where the injury occurred. This is all done through a finely tuned system that constantly adjusts pressure based on the needs of your body (Pober & Sessa, 2015).

The juxtaposition occurs because, unlike when you are "in the mood" for sex, when you have an acute injury, like a sprained ankle, the increase in sensitivity to touch isn't pleasurable. It's painful. Same mechanism (increased blood flow), but the output is very different.

The output that is movement requires two things: expansion and compression. These are complementary pairs, dependent on each other for the generation of movement. Expansion and compression happens throughout the body, creating pressure in places like at the ribs or in a joint.

In order to better understand this, I asked Adarian what expansion and compression meant. During the course of our friendship, he has taken on the arduous task of breaking down complex concepts so that I can actually understand them and disseminate them in written format. (For those of you wondering, this takes the patience of some sort of otherworldly being—I ask enough questions to put a curious four-year-old to shame.)

Adarian broke it down like this: Imagine a balloon. When you blow up the balloon, it is expanding without compression. When the balloon is deflating it is compressing without expansion.

In the body, compression without expansion leads to folding. Imagine a diver tucked in a ball as they turn through the air. Without expansion, they won't be able to slow down and control their entry into the water.

Expansion without compression is like a void. If that same diver sprawled their body out with nothing internally compressing their torso, when they hit the water there will be nothing to prevent them from breaking.

So you need both, and the one force that is constantly acting on the body, allowing this internal pressure to go up and down, is gravity.

Complementary pairs, because it takes two to tango:

When pressure is applied to the skin, the skin gently deforms, compressing. But it also expands outward, acquiescing to the increased pressure. When your partner leans into you and you respond by leaning into them, you are compressing, but for something to compress, something else has to expand, somewhere.

As soon as the pressure against the skin is released, it expands to its original shape, and as your partner leans away from you, you either lean into them more to recreate the sense of compression or you expand up and away from them.

When you establish closeness with someone, there is a gentle back and forth of compression and expansion as you search for the desired amount of contact. One may be more prevalent than the other at certain times as you arch back or coil in, but both are involved to achieve just the right amount of connection and space.

Movement is no different. When I run, I generate internal pressure and compression as my foot lands and my body moves down. As my leg straightens and extends behind me, I stand up, creating tension through expansion. Tension refers to the pulling that occurs on the soft tissue when things are tightly stretched. It's the tension that allows you to move quickly, returning to a position where there is less compression and pressure. When I deadlift a heavy weight, I compress, creating a high amount of internal pressure to pick up the bar; as I stand up, I create tension to allow my body to expand.

Compression is the result of pressure; expansion is the result of tension. The interplay between compression, pressure, expansion, and tension are what allow me to transition from one position to another. Which means it should make sense that when I roll around on the floor, tucking myself into a ball and reaching out of the ball, the compression allows me to create contact while the expansion generates movement. The compression complements the expansion and the expansion complements the compression.

The internal pressure you create allows you to generate input. When you use that input to push away from the ground, what force is acting on you to pull you back down to the ground? The force that made Sir Isaac Newton ponder why apples never fall sideways—they only fall straight down to the ground. And that force is a universal constant everyone living on earth has to find a way to navigate: gravity.

Gravity: A lifelong love affair

You enter the world after incubating for (usually) nine months surrounded by the fluid of your mother's womb, intimately connected to your mother. She is your life force, providing nutrients and the warm environment in which you float.

You enter the world violently, exiting your safe cocoon and trading it in for a world where you are no longer floating. Instead, you are forced to overcome the constant pull of the earth, hurling your body through space in an attempt to generate movement.

During your first year, you figure out how to move farther and farther away from the ground. The force of gravity is constantly pulling you back down, only for you to totter back up, uncertainly at first, but as time goes on, more and more confidently.

By the time you are an adult, the ground is no longer a place you spend much time. The constant pull of the earth is something that is navigated without thought—unless you fall—and then you find yourself thinking how much the ground hurts.

When you learn how to use gravity to your advantage so you can create more input, there is an increase of sensations in different places, changing how you use your joints, your muscles, and your body. This can turn up sensation in certain areas and dial it down in others.

Gravity isn't something to fear. It's something that increases your output by giving you input. It's the partner you dance with every single day as you move through the world. You might as well make the dance a reciprocating one so that you get to lead occasionally.

You can alter your relationship with gravity a number of ways. Learning to befriend gravity is a way to create compression through your joints and body; learning to push away from gravity enables you to expand out into space.

You furl and unfurl, coil and uncoil, with every move as you and gravity take turns leading. Think about various movements that you do on a regular basis. You bend and extend when you walk or get up and sit down in a chair. You squat down and extend up when you jump. If you want to spin fast, you coil in; if you want to spin slowly, you expand out.

This lifelong love affair can be passionate. Sometimes gravity pulls forcefully, insisting you yield your entire structure as you relent to the ground.

But sometimes it's a gentle nudge, reminding you to yield so that you don't break. The nudges serve as opportunities to dance a little bit differently.

A lesson in self-directed pressure:

How do you learn to create internal pressure so that you and gravity can enjoy a lifelong partnership? Let's start by looking at something that generates internal pressure, compression, and expansion every single day: the breath.

When you inhale, air enters the body through the nose or mouth, moves into the lungs where oxygen is extracted and then out into the blood. The lungs are sponge-like and can't actually expand on their own. Remember that expansion and compression work together in the body, so it might not be surprising that lungs expand because the muscles in the chest and abdomen contract, creating a vacuum-like action around the lungs so air can flow in. Another way to think of this: the compression of the muscles against the lungs allow the lungs to expand.

The oxygen extracted from the air is able to move from outside of the body into the bloodstream through a series of pressure changes. Air is a gas, and gases move from high-pressure areas to low-pressure areas. The air that you breathe is no exception; moving from the relative high-pressure of the atmosphere and into the lungs, which are comprised of tiny air sacs called alveoli. (Don't worry. There is no quiz. The technical terms are for illustration only.) This increases the pressure in the lungs, which causes the air to move into the space between them, a.k.a. the pleural cavity (Charalampidis et al., 2015).

When you exhale, you create a vacuum in the pleural cavity, just like the piston does on the fuel mixture in the car engine, as the muscles of breathing relax. This increases intra-alveolar pressure, which pushes air out of the lungs and back into the world. The exhale creates the spark.

To put this more simply: air comes in; muscles compress lungs; lungs expand; rib cage expands; organs move down; oxygen moves from lungs to pleural cavity and into blood stream.

Then: Muscles relax; lungs compress; rib cage gets smaller; organs move up; air moves from lung space to lungs and into the atmosphere.

Or, as Adarian puts it, "as you move, you breathe."

Another term for this is locomotion-respiratory coupling. This refers to the breathing and stepping rhythms that occurs in several vertebrates (including humans). When a horse gallops, for instance, the breathing-stepping rhythm is 1:1—one breath per each step (Daley et al., 2013).

Humans show more variability, sometimes taking one breath for every two steps, or one breath for every four steps; and sometimes there is no discernible rhythm between stepping and breathing at all. It's been suggested that having a rhythmic relationship between breathing and stepping during walking and running minimizes loading in the breathing muscles, makes breathing easier and minimizing fatigue. Basically, it's a positive thing when locomotion-respiratory coupling occurs.

Every single inhale and exhale you take leads to a sequence of events because of air coming in and air going out. Which variables can you alter to change your experience of breathing?

You can change the speed at which you inhale or exhale. You can change how you are inhaling or exhaling by directing your inhale into your mid-back or your chest or your lateral rib cage. You can change when you inhale or when you exhale.

Containing vibrations:

When you land on the ground, there is a jolt that echos through your body. How loud the jolt is depends on how you contain the jolt.

The jolt is a vibration, a back and forth movement of particles in the body that occur whenever the body is knocked off-center (which occurs whenever you move). Vibration is what allows you to restore your equilibrium by responding to the forces acting upon you (Encyclopedia Britannica, 2022).

Vibration, then, is the sense of reverb that echos through your body, the subtle hum of energy that becomes a nuanced soundtrack as you move, contracting and expanding.

Vibration can be aurally pleasing. It can meet the ears and immediately be absorbed as you translate the vibration to movement.

Or it can feel jarring, like a sudden jolt of unwanted energy moving through your system with nowhere to go, bringing you to an abrupt stop.

When you hit your funny bone against something, the impact echos through your elbow, down into your hand. It jolts you, causing an unpleasant sensation that makes your bones vibrate.

Another way to think of a vibration is that it is what happens as the result of a collision between your body and something else. Some collisions are desirable, pleasurable even. Others threaten your physical sense of safety and well-being. But the body, in its infinite wisdom, has ways to turn the unwanted vibrations that are the result of the collision into ones that are wanted and beneficial to the entire structure. This happens through pressure, which harnesses the vibration's impact and turns it into something powerful.

Every single time you move, there is vibration through your body at the cellular level. The bigger the vibration, the more noise deep within you responds.

Think about osteoporosis, a common bone disease associated with aging. During osteoporosis, the innermost part of the bone changes. It literally means "porous bone" because the structural changes make the bone weak and susceptible to injury (Porter & Varacallo, 2022).

But (and here's where things get interesting), it turns out if you want to stimulate the cells of the bone to grow, you need to add high-vibration stress (Bacabac et al., 2006). One way to do that is through external collisions.

Internal and external collisions: Fast and furious or slow and laborious

Collisions are a critical aspect of movement; in fact, they are movement, when you consider every single move you make sets off the subtlest vibration throughout your entire system.

To put this more simply: collisions cause vibrations.

When the vibrations that occur because of the collision are unwanted and you don't have the ability to turn them into wanted vibrations, the internal sound that results is like the sound of a car with an engine that isn't functioning properly. It might be subtly annoying at first, gradually getting louder until you can't stand it any longer. Or it might happen suddenly, as you are driving down the street and you suddenly hear a loud wheezing noise that causes you to think, uh oh. That's not good.

In your car, this generally means you need to take it to a mechanic and have it assessed and repaired so you can continue driving it without fear of ending up on the side of the road. The body really isn't that different. If you pay attention to the soft, irritating vibrations before they become loud, you can easily change how you are vibrating and make things hum along smoothly again. If you ignore the sound for too long, it becomes a much bigger issue and your body, just like your car, won't perform as well.

And sometimes life brings big collisions that lead to big unwanted vibrations. The resulting injury might require time before the impact from the unwanted vibrations becomes quieter, and the gentle, pleasant thrumming noise you are accustomed to returns.

Adarian explains it like this, "Every impact is a collision. Every movement is a way to manage the collision. If your goal is high-level performance, you want to create the collision, not let it happen to you. The thing that differentiates the two is the speed."

What happens at impact determines whether the vibration is wanted or unwanted. Do you arch up into it? Shift your torso towards it? Rock away from it?

Consider a boxer being struck by another boxer's fist. The blow is undesired. The impact creates a ripple through the entire body.

How that ripple is felt and experienced depends on the way the boxer takes the hit. Do they lean into it, acquiescing to the vibration in the same way the skin acquiesced to pressure earlier? Or do they lean away, attempting to avoid the inevitable jolt?

It might seem counterintuitive, but if the boxer leans away, attempting to avoid the impact, their system won't know what to do with the unwanted vibration from the experience of the collision. And when the boxer's entire body seems to come to a halt, their body against the floor of the ring, the sense of ringing in their body will take a long time to cease.

But what about the boxer who leans into the collision, allowing the force to move through their body? How does this change things?

Leaning in allows the boxer to yield to the impact rather than brace for it. To yield means to surrender or submit; by leaning in, the boxer surrenders to the collision and the vibrations echo through their body in a softer way, making the unwanted, wanted. Or at least, tolerated.

Since collisions are going to occur regardless of what you do, you might as well learn to manage them and make resulting vibrations wanted.

Adarian says there are controlled and uncontrolled collisions. Controlled collisions create wanted vibrations.

Think of a child on a swing. When you time the push just right, the child benefits from the enjoyment of a smooth ride up, and a smooth ride down. The child smiles, maybe even laughs gleefully, asking for the pushing to continue. The child is experiencing a wanted collision.

But what if the timing of the push isn't very good? The child's swing up and down is jarring. The child becomes unhappy and wants to get off. The collision is no longer wanted and the resulting vibration is unpleasant.

Navigating collisions is tricky. There will be times when collisions happen unexpectedly, like when you find yourself falling uncontrollably or you realize someone's fist is coming at you too fast to react. But if you learn to manage the collision and lean into it a little bit, you can make the unwanted, wanted.

Internal balance: A dynamic act

When you search for the seemingly elusive quality of elation, that exquisite sense of freedom that comes from successfully channeling vibrations into something that is wanted creates a lightness. There is this moment when it's as though everything within you is perfectly harmonious and calm, yet ready for whatever collision comes next. This moment is balance.

Homeostasis is a term that refers to the ever-changing landscape within you. It's a constant, dynamic process that is always occurring, keeping an internal sense of balance among your cells, your organs, and the rest of you as you move through the world. It's a self-regulatory process that allows you to adapt and survive while being challenged. It allows your heart rate to spike when you lift something heavy, only for your heart rate to return to its normal resting rhythm when you stop. It's the reason you can go run in ninty-five degree weather; even though the outside air feels hot, your body cools itself down by sweating so your internal temperature doesn't elevate. When you stop running, it takes a minute for the system to realize you are no longer performing vigorous activity. Once it does, the sweating stops.

Without homeostasis, you would be in constant threat of disease, injury, and being unable to adapt to the environment around you. Balance reduces physiological threat. Imbalance creates vulnerability. Homeostasis is the art of internal balance (Billman, 2020).

Every single concept we've discussed so far is a way for the system (you) to maintain homeostasis. Expansion. Compression. Pressure. Collisions. Vibrations. All of these things work together to create balance. The input that affects how these five words are expressed comes from you—how do you vibrate? How do you navigate collisions? The output is the movement.

CHAPTER 2

YOU ARE THE MOVEMENT

There is this moment, when you shift just a little, to increase pressure because the pressure increases sensation. First you try shifting your right hip. When that doesn't work, you reach your left shoulder blade down, seeking for just the right spot to find that moment of balanced pressure, balanced sensation.

Elation, remember, is that moment of movement freedom and balance. It is created when the right amount of pressure is applied to create the desired response. The application of pressure is input; the desired response is output. That sweet spot is determined by position.

If the pressure applied doesn't lead to the desired output, you have the power to change how you apply the pressure. And the power you have is based on position, which is based on compression and expansion.

Position is the culmination of your joints. It is determined by the angles at which the joints are bent and how much compression and expansion are occurring at each joint. If you want to find the optimal position to accomplish a task, you need to learn how to navigate the levers that are your body.

The example Adarian gave me when I asked him how position relates to levers is this:

> Imagine you are getting ready to open a tight-lidded jar. What do you do?

You brace and twist the lid with the positioned hand. The hand is the lever; you optimize the use of the hand as a lever by the position of you body.

What this means is even the slightest shift in position will affect the way you are using levers to move. This gives you the ultimate power—if you can feel your position, you can change your position. Changing your position changes pressure and changing pressure changes your movement.

Imagine this: what if I told you you could make an exercise like a push-up feel easy, light even? Would that be more interesting than push-ups that feel miserable?

Or that you could run in a way that felt more effortless than effortful, a way that felt fast and smooth?

Or that you when you felt a niggle of sensation somewhere, you could make a small shift away from the pressure and the niggle might dissipate? Or that if you were seeking sensation, you could shift into it, applying more pressure and increasing the pleasurable experience?

All of these things, and more, are possible with a basic understanding of how levers work. So let's dive into how you can achieve movement freedom.

An overview of levers:

Every single time you move, your body shifts. Your muscles strain, pulling bones in a way that produces movement. How you shift depends on a variety of factors, including how you've moved before, what you "think" the desired outcome is, and how you are currently navigating pressure, compression, and expansion.

This coordination and the movement that results are based on three different axes of rotation: pitch, yaw, and roll. We will cover these concepts more thoroughly in chapters 3 and 6, but for now, consider this:

Pitch can either act by itself, with yaw or roll, or with yaw and roll. The same is true for yaw and roll. So rotation is either based on a singular axis, like a bike tire rotating in a straight line, or it can be more complex, like a top trying to remain upright.

As I mentioned earlier, your brain is constantly getting information from your body regarding its location in space. That's because of specialized cells called mechanoreceptors that detect touch, pressure, vibration, and sound from their internal and external environment (French & Torkkeli, 2009).

There is a term for this sense your brain has about the body's position. It's called proprioception and it's unconscious. You always have this underlying sense of where your body is and how your joints are bent even if you don't realize it, and that's because of the pressure the brain detects.

Imagine you're on a sports team, and your coach makes a suggestion to try a specific movement a different way. So you make the suggested change, or at least you think you make the suggested change, and the coach comes over and gently says, "okay, now can you try it with your left knee bent?"

"My left knee is bent," you reply, wondering what's wrong with your coach's eyes.

The coach whips out their cell phone and says, "let's film it and see. Try it one more time."

So you do the exercise one more time, certain your left knee is bent so far your leg is bent in half. When you watch the video playback you realize that not only is your left knee not bent as much as you thought it was, it's barely bent at all.

Your perception of your body and its parts doesn't always match what's actually happening. And that's because the image your brain has of your body, a.k.a. your body schema or your body map, is updated based on the input the brain receives from your peripheral nervous system, the part of the nervous system that's in charge of all things body related.

If you don't ever take the time to fine-tune your detection of the input or the input itself, there will be a mismatch between perception and reality. You can update your body map through focused attention. In other words, you can update your perception through mindful movement. In fact, we've included an exercise chapter later in the book that can help fold this science into your workouts.

In the meantime, consider this: touch is a form of pressure. Sound is a form of vibration. Input is based on pressure and vibration. Pressure is based on compression and expansion. Vibration occurs at the cellular level and is based on your response to collisions.

These cells are sensitive. They notice when you change position slowly. They notice when you change position quickly. They sense the subtlest shift in pressure. Every time you compress a little more, moving towards something, or expand slightly, moving away from something, those cells send electrical signals up to your brain. Input creates an electrical charge. A vibration (Ergen & Ulkar, 2009).

The creation of position:

A lever is a simple machine that consists of a fulcrum and a lever arm. A fulcrum is a pivot point, the support about which a lever moves. Random fact: according to Merriam-Webster (n.d.), the word fulcrum means "bedpost" in Latin and means "to prop."

To put it more simply: the fulcrum supports the part that is moving.

You can also think of the fulcrum as the end of an anchor. It is the pivot point, the place rotation occurs.

Levers exist to make it easier to manipulate a load. You use levers to let something heavy down gently. Or to lift up something heavy.

The effort to do this comes from you. Whether it is easy or hard to move the load depends on where effort is applied on the lever arm to create movement around the fulcrum. We will discuss this in further detail in chapter 5 when we talk about complementary pairs.

Lift your arm straight out in front of you. Which part is the lever and which part is the fulcrum?

The arm and fingertips are the lever arm. The shoulder is the fulcrum.

What is the load? The arm and fingers.

What allows the lever to lift? How do the fingers move from next to your body to straight out in front of you? Through effort that is exerted by the muscles in the shoulder. Or the muscles in the scapula. Why? Because how you use your body depends on where your fulcrum is located.

If you want to move the arm faster, what can you do?

Bend the elbow. This shortens the lever arm.

If you want to make the arm move slower, what do you do?

Hold on to something that extends the lever arm, like a broomstick.

If you want to shift the fulcrum point from the shoulder to the shoulder blade, what do you do?

Consciously change how you are doing the movement by allowing the shoulder blade to participate in the lifting.

But wait, what is a lever?

Right about here, I got confused. I understood a lever produced movement. It was a simple machine consisting of a fulcrum and a lever arm. But in the context of movement and, more specifically, human movement, what is a lever?

The answer, according to Adarian, is you. You are a collection of simple machines, of fulcrums and lever arms that produce movement. How you produce movement depends on your position because the input is the output.

To make things more interesting, when the input ends the output ends.

Think about this for a second: the output (in our case, movement), only lasts as long as the input does.

Let's consider our juxtaposition from the last chapter: pleasure and pain. When you apply pressure that is experienced in a pleasurable way, the pleasure only lasts as long as the pressure does. On the other hand, if you apply pressure that is painful to a specific area, the experience of pain will last only as long as the pressure does. The input is the output.

Pretend you are doing a deadlift. There is pressure applied to your torso via compression as you lift the weight off the ground. What allows you to lift the weight off the ground? Levers. What is the lever in this situation? The torso. What is the load? The barbell. Where is the fulcrum? The hips. Where does the effort come from to overcome the load of the barbell? The muscles in the torso.

When you finish the lift, what happens? (We talked about this a little bit last chapter.) The compression changes. Your position is different. The weight will feel less heavy when you are holding it in a standing position than it did when you were picking it up off the floor. Why? The input is different so the output is different because your position changed.

Believe it or not, this is an easy example. Whenever you have an external load, like a barbell, the lever is going to be more straightforward. How you use your body to lift the load is related to extrinsic properties, including the tactile information you receive from the object, like whether your fingers detect the object is hard or soft, smooth or rough, warm or cool. This information helps your brain create a picture of the tool you are using, which it then adopts into its vision of you (Sun & Tang, 2019). This input informs your output, and while you can change things that will impact how efficient the lever is like the position of your torso in relation to your legs or the position of your legs in relation to your torso, for the most part, the motion is relatively fixed.

When you consider a movement like running, everything is more internal. You are the source of the input, rather than an external barbell.

To make matters more interesting, when you run, the lever is constantly shifting as you move through space. You start on your left foot as your right foot swings through the air. Your shoulder blades may or may not compress, depending on what's happening at the foot. The right foot lands, transferring the weight over to the right leg. Depending on what happened in the right foot, the upper body may or may not rotate.

But the levers that allow the movement of running are no different than the levers that allow the movement of dead lifting. They are still coming from you. Let's break this down further.

Pretend you are walking. Imagine that moment when the left foot hits the ground. It anchors you briefly as your body moves up and over it. The lever arm, in this case, is the foot that's in contact with the ground. The fulcrum is the ankle joint. The load is the weight of your body and gravity. The effort comes from the muscles around the ankle joint.

As your left foot comes in contact with the ground, the right leg swings back and propels itself forward. How does this happen? Because of the fulcrum that is the right hip. The lever arm is the right leg. The load is also the right leg. The effort comes from the muscles around the hip.

You can change the sequencing of the levers by altering your position. If you lean back when the left foot is in contact with the ground, you put the brakes on, increasing the length of the collision that occurs between the foot and the ground. If you pull the right foot off the ground when the left foot makes contact, the effort comes from the right hamstring instead of the right gluteal muscle, changing how you use the right leg as a lever.

Hold on, you might be thinking, this is a lot to keep track of, and why do I even care? The answer is based on one of the main points from last chapter: because if you understand what the levers are and where the fulcrum is, you can manage your collisions rather than let collisions happen to you.

The art of collisions:

Imagine you are catching your partner. They extend towards you. You alter your body position slightly to catch them gently.

As you hold them, you prepare to move them away from you, back to the ground. Your body shifts again, so you can create a sense of stability, a strong base of support so they can feel safe on their journey away from you.

Now imagine you are the one being caught and thrown. As you feel yourself moving towards your partner, you soften, trusting that the arms about to encompass you will pull you in rather than push you away.

After that brief moment of safety, you feel your partner's position shift, preparing to push you out and away. You feel an internal sense of strength as you fly through the air, softening again as you impact with the floor.

Levers are a way to explore movement as an act of catching and launching. You receive the ground, you leave the ground. How you do that is based on how you use your body; how you anchor yourself, how you bend, where you bend from. Once you begin to identify these things, if there's something you want, like more pressure, more speed, or more control, you have the power to change the input. And what happens when you change the input? How you organize your levers changes because, as Adarian likes to say, "the input is the output."

What feels better? Receiving a kiss straight on, or rotating the head a little bit as the lips meet? What about when you are about to be caught by your partner? Do you rotate your body into them as they are receiving you? Or do you keep your body oriented straight ahead as they try to bring you into them?

Rarely does impact feel best when it's dealt with head on, without any rotation at all. Rotation allows you to shorten the collision so you can keep moving forward in space; if a gymnast is in the middle of their tumbling routine, performing one trick after another, they want the collision to be short so they can maintain momentum.

Rotation can also allow you to extend the collision so you can linger, pausing in the moment. Do you want to hurry the kiss or extend the kiss? These choices impact how you deal with the vibrations that occur as a result of the collision, allowing you to move fast or slow, sharply or sensitively.

This idea of rotation as a way to deal with collisions is conveniently built into the lever system that is your body. A critical aspect of understanding movement is grasping that every movement is a rotation; in order for a lever to move, rotation occurs at the fulcrum *even in movements that look like they are happening in a linear, or straight, way.*

Rotation occurs when the lever arm is perpendicular to the fulcrum and compression is applied at the fulcrum so a parallel effort can be exerted. The parallel creates the rotation. The compression creates the connection.

Think about this: you are performing the dead lift from earlier. It looks like the bar comes straight off the ground because your torso moves straight back in space. The hips move back so you can grab the bar, the hips move forward so you can pick up the bar.

In order for this to happen, the torso moves back so the shoulders are perpendicular to the bar. Have you ever tried to dead lift with the barbell in front of the shoulders? It doesn't feel great, mostly because it feels a lot harder. What about with the shoulders in front of the barbell?

While this is a great way to make the movement feel harder, it doesn't exactly make you feel beast-mode strong.

Parallels and perpendiculars need each other. They are complementary pairs. The perpendicular allows compression throughout the torso and hips. This compression creates an opportunity for the lever to work efficiently.

The parallel and perpendicular also create the rotation that occurs during movement.

The body, of course, operates at more than just right angles. So it isn't necessarily the angle of the joint that is perpendicular. It's how input is being applied to create compression.

The fulcrum of the barbell dead lift, which is the hips, aren't moving just front and back. They are rotating up and over the leg. This allows you, as Adarian says, to not run into yourself.

Have you ever put together furniture using a hex wrench? When you insert the hex wrench into the screw, you turn the wrench. Why? Because this turns the screw. Or, more accurately, this rotates the screw. The entire goal of using a hex wrench is to rotate the screw so it can connect two stable objects together so they form an angle.

In order for the hex wrench to turn the screw, the lever arm (which is the hex wrench) is perpendicular to the screw. You then gently push the wrench into the screw before you begin rotating the screw. You compress in order to rotate.

The force you apply to rotate the wrench is parallel to the fulcrum between the screw and the hex wrench. The fulcrum in this example is the axis of rotation. If the force weren't applied parallel to the axis of rotation, the wrench would slip out of the screw.

In a movement like a dead lift, the hips compress before you lift the barbell off the ground, creating a more effective connection between the fulcrum and the lever arm. The muscles are then able to rotate you up with a force that is again applied parallel to the axis of rotation.

Where is the axis of rotation in this example? At the hip joint.

Class III lever

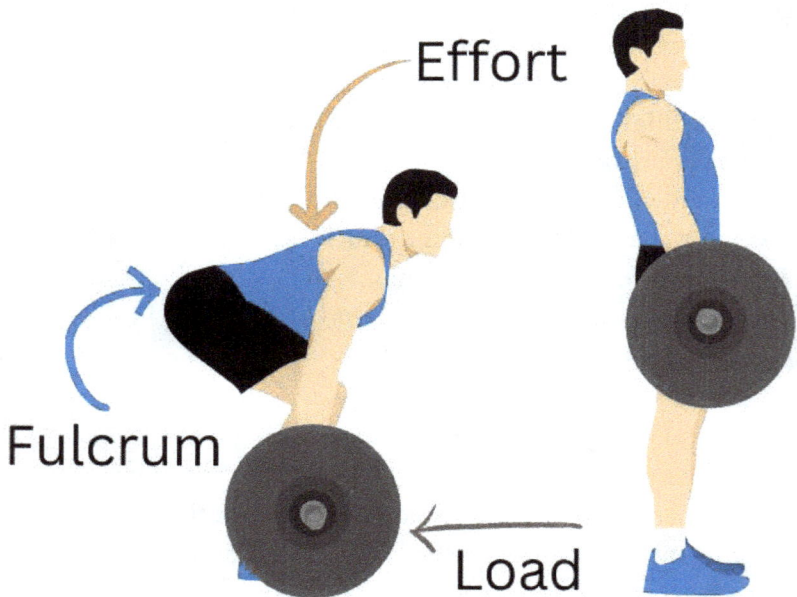

Effort

Fulcrum

Load

Next time you are doing a dead lift, try this: As you set up with the bar, imagine the hips are the axis of rotation. As you are standing up, feel your torso rotating around the hips. Does that change how you experience the movement?

Do you remember what the goal of a lever is during movement?

To make it easier to move.

And if it's easier to move, what happens?

It's more enjoyable to do the things that you want to do and it's easier to access strength, mobility, and speed.

Remember when I asked whether it felt better to receive a kiss straight on or with the head rotated slightly? If both people come at each other head-on, they run into each other. So instead, both people rotate. This enables them to establish just the right amount of pressure as their lips connect.

When you begin looking at movement through the lens of identifying a fulcrum and lever arm, you are also identifying where the axis of rotation happens. Regardless of whether you are navigating an external load or creating internally generated movement, you are rotating. As Adarian says, "Linear will lead you wrong all day long."

The thing that allows you to rotate is the collision. How you navigate the collision creates the rotations that move you forward.

When you look at something many people do regularly, like run, being able to see the rotations becomes a valuable source of information. You can think of running as four different rotations broken down like this:

The right ankle, which is acting as a class-one lever, rotates as the foot hits the ground. (See the appendix for a quick breakdown of the three different types of levers.)

The left glute lifts.

The obliques rotate the torso to the left.

The left scapula compresses and rotates to the left.

This is theoretical. Often what happens is the right ankle doesn't rotate. Or the obliques don't rotate the torso to the left. Or the left scapula doesn't compress.

And when any of the above things happen, they affect the other levers. Remember, the input is the output. Change any internal input and the output changes.

Earlier, I mentioned levers can make a push-up easier. Let's look at how that works.

What is the lever arm in a push-up? The torso.

What is the fulcrum? The knees or feet.

What is the load? The torso.

Where is the effort? In the arms.

Given this information, what can you do to make a push-up easier?

You can change the load by changing the position of the torso. This can look like elevating the hands, shifting the torso back, or coming onto the knees.

If you feel pretty good about push-ups in a regular position, what can you focus on to make your push-up feel easier?

You can make sure the torso is stiff. Why? It's easier to move something that is more rigid than it is to move something less rigid.

Imagine you have to move a mattress that weighs forty-five pounds and a weight plate that weighs forty-five pounds. Which is going to be easier to move?

The weight plate. Not only is it a less cumbersome size, it's a solid object. The mattress is sloppy, awkward to move from point A to point B.

What else will make the push-up easier?

Try thinking about pulling yourself down with your hands or imagining the muscles around the shoulder blade are pulling the torso down, and then pushing the arms straight.

When you understand the lever, you begin determining what you are doing, how you are doing it, and when you are doing it. And these three things are the keys to athletic movement. "Assess the levers," Adarian told me once. The rest takes care of itself.

CHAPTER 3

THE ART AND SCIENCE OF MOVING

You thrust your hips up, looking for that specific sensation, the one that indicates you are on the right path: the path to deep inner connection.

As you lower them down, you focus, your intention on the next thrust up, the one that will bring you closer to what you are seeking, the freedom of a flexible and strong pelvis, a pelvis that allows you to perform in all areas of your life.

Movement elation is predicated on the ability of the body to move a variety of ways. The pelvis is the place where the center of mass is located (for most people), which means moving it alters your sense of center. It's where your leg connects to your torso and where your torso ends.

It's also the place we associate with sexual pleasure, birthing a child, and the expulsion of waste from the body. Needless to say, there are a lot of ideas surrounding the pelvis and its role in, well, just about everything related to moving. One thing most experts agree on is that the muscles surrounding the pelvis should be strong and flexible.

Levers and hips: A practical example

Enter the hip thrust, an exercise that is heralded to increase gluteal strength. It's supposed to make you strong, make your backside perky, and give you unparalleled booty strength so you can sprint and jump. This makes it a go-to for everyone in the weight room. They place their upper backs on benches, their feet strongly rooted to the floor. A barbell is placed across their hips as they lower them towards the ground and push their hips back up, one rep after another.

This is an excellent example of an exercise that promises one thing, but is actually a poor use of the way that specific lever works. The hip thrust promises gluteus maximus strength; but, the gluteus maximus is a big muscle, one that is, according to one anatomy text, quadrangular shaped. I had to look up what a quadrangle was. It turns out, it's a four-sided plane figure that looks something like this shadow:

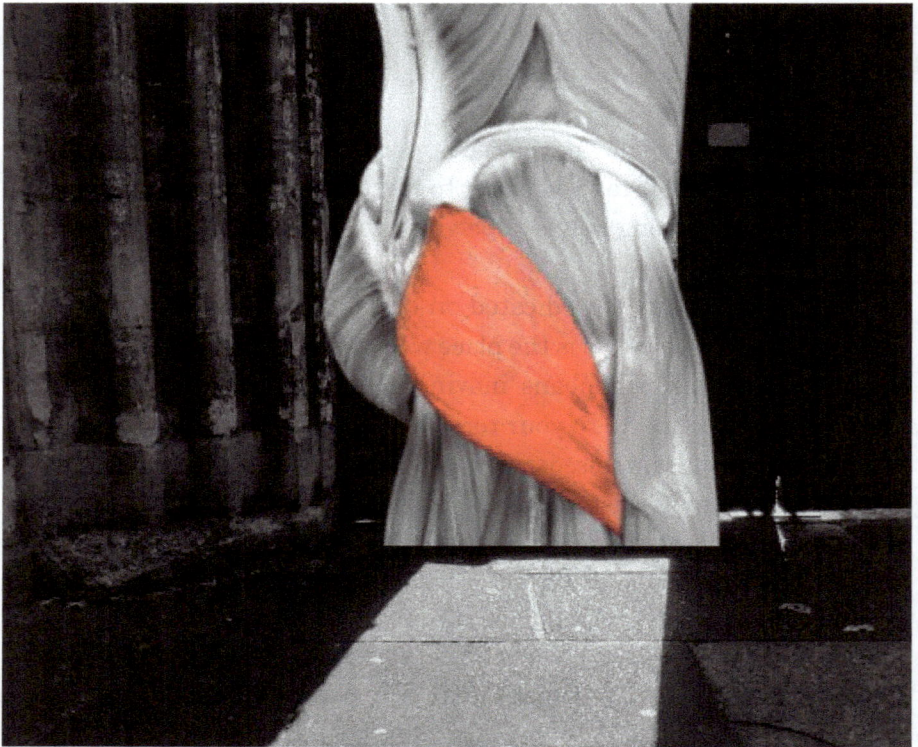

PHOTO BY JAMES WAINSCOAT ON UNSPLASH

The gluteus maximus attaches to several bony areas, including the pelvis, low-back, and femur (the long thigh bone). It depends on the position of the torso for the gluteus maximus to act as an efficient lever to pull and rotate the thigh bone.

I said earlier that there are three axes of rotation that can act either alone or in conjunction with one (or both) of the other axes. Those axes of rotation are pitch, yaw, and roll. How rotation occurs at each joint depends on the muscles that cross those joints.

If a muscle only affects one axis of rotation, it can be thought of as a 1D muscle. If it affects two axes of rotation, it is a 2D muscle.

Muscles that cross joints either create a drawing in, a compression that secures the bone in the socket, or they pull the bones away from the body, creating an expansion of the limb through space.

The short head of the biceps brachii, for instance, which is one of the pop-eye muscles that flexes the elbow, draws the forearm towards the upper arm. The elbow bones around the elbow joint fold, decreasing the appearance of length at the upper limb.

The medial head of the triceps brachii, which is one of the muscles that extends the elbow, brings the upper arm and the lower arm away from each other. The arm expands, becoming long (Hussain et al., 2020).

When a muscle crosses two joints, it's considered a biarticular muscle. Both the biceps brachii and the triceps brachii are actually biarticular muscles, which means they affect two different joints, the shoulder and the elbow. They allow rotation to happen, and prevent too much twisting from happening at the joint. Biarticular muscles keep joints safe from too much strain. We've talked only about the elbow joint to keep things simple, but later on the concept of biarticular muscles will be important.

The gluteus maximus is a 2D muscle, affecting two axes of rotation at the hip: pitch and yaw, or the extension of the thigh back and the rotation of the thigh out, away from midline. The effectiveness of the gluteus maximus as a 2D muscle depends on a number of things, including position of the leg and position of the torso.

Now that you have a general understanding of muscles and movement, let's get back to looking at the hip thrust, an exercise that, according to some of the research, is no more effective at isolating the muscles in the back of the leg than the Romanian dead lift or step up (Delgado et al., 2019; Neto et al., 2020). Look at the picture of the hip thrust below. What is the fulcrum?

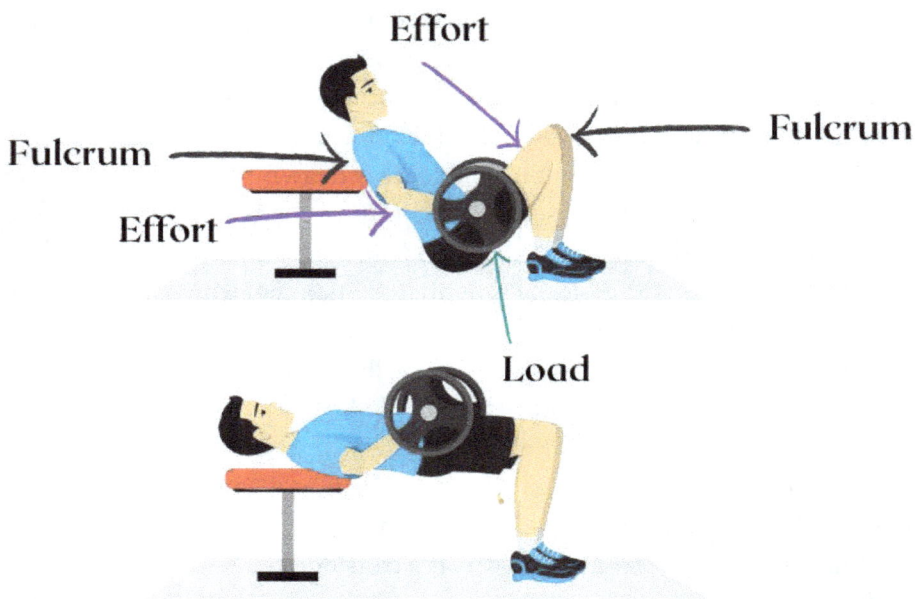

Class III levers

There are two: at the shoulder that is on the bench and at the knee joint if the shin is vertical.

Here's where things get really interesting when you are assessing levers. The levers lifting the weight up aren't the gluteal muscles. They are the torso and the thighs.

Let's take this a step further. When the gluteus maximus is functioning as a class-three lever, it's either working to create strength or range during a hip extension. If you are using the hip thrust to make your gluteus maximus stronger for activities like running or jumping, is this an effective way to train how that muscle functions as a lever?

No, since it isn't even the lever that is being used to accomplish the motion.

Let that sink in for a second. It's commonly taught that the gluteus maximus is the primary lever that is being used to lift the torso, but it isn't.

So does the hip thrust translate to gluteus maximus speed that will help you while running or jumping? Probably not. How well the gluteus maximus is working as a lever during more athletic movement depends on a variety of factors, including your shin angle (which we will discuss in chapter 5) and your torso position.

What else does the hip thrust resemble? A movement that is often found in the bedroom, but get this—it's not exactly great for that, either. Why? Think about collisions. Think about rotations. Think about what you have learned so far about collisions and rotations. Straight-on collisions cause unwanted vibrations. Rotation makes things wanted.

The gluteus maximus acts as a lever arm for movement at the hip by generating rotation at the hip joint. This rotation allows the leg to move behind you. So if you want to effectively target the gluteus maximus, you need to target the action of hip rotation. The hip needs to be the fulcrum for movement.

Check out the example below. Can you identify the lever and the fulcrum?

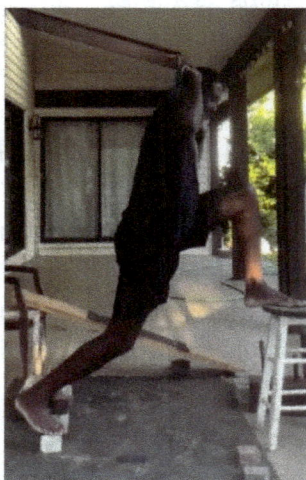 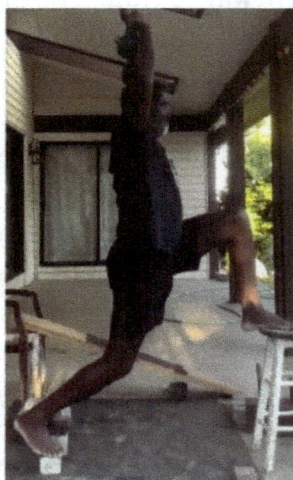

Start   Finish

I used the hip thrust as an example, but once you understand levers, you can apply this type of critical thinking to any movement. Is the hip thrust a bad exercise? No. There aren't any "bad exercises." But does it accomplish what it is marketed as doing? I will let you be the one to decide.

Compress to move:

When you coil or compress in, you create pressure. This compression allows you to control your position. You can shift towards something, move away from something, explode out of something, or gently glide into something, all while maintaining a sense of control. Control is a by-product of moving easily, efficiently.

You also learned a few pages back that compression allows you to rotate. When two lips meet, they establish connection via compression before more movement takes place. The set up (heads rotate, lips meet) determines what happens next.

And this is true of all movements. Remember, the input is the output. The set up creates what happens next.

For the purposes of this book, we are going to put muscles in two groups: muscles that compress and muscles that act as lever arms. Some, like the obliques, can be either a lever arm or can create compression. It's an either/or situation: they can't be both a lever arm and provide compression at the same time.

Another way to think about the importance of creating compression is that it allows you to create collisions. "I've got to create a collision to create the energy to keep me moving," Adarian told me.

And this, for those of you who have taken a physics class, should make a little bit of sense. Energy is in a constant state of flux. It's transferred from potential energy, or inert energy, to kinetic energy, or movement. In the body, this works like this:

- There is a specialized form of chemical energy that lives in your cells called adenosine triphosphate (ATP). Unlike bitcoin, it can be thought of as actual currency, like cash.

- When ATP isn't being used, it gets saved in a rainy day fund.

- Once you begin moving, muscular contractions require energy, so the chemical energy of ATP gets converted to mechanical work, a.k.a. kinetic energy, that the cells use to fuel the contractions.

- When movement or muscular contraction stops, the rainy day account builds itself back up by generating more ATP as chemical energy (Dunn & Grider, 2022).

When Adarian talks about creating energy he is referring to that shift of potential, unharnessed energy to energy that is being harnessed to move you forward. The chemical energy that is ATP becomes the kinetic energy that is movement.

Because this isn't an anatomy book, I am not going to go into detail about the different muscles, where they are located, and their actions. Just know this: if you look at a picture of a muscle, if there are several muscles underneath it, there is a good chance it acts like a lever arm. If the muscle lies deep, underneath other muscles, there is a good chance it provides compression.

In the hip joint (since we just did an entire review of the hip thrust), the muscles underneath the gluteus maximus are the gluteus medius and gluteus minimus; there are also six smaller muscles that surround the hip joint itself (these are often called the deep six or the rotator cuff of the hip). These muscles all provide compression to the hip joint and pelvis.

You can also think of these muscles as anchoring the hip to the pelvis. Anchoring (and compression) are what provide input about where body parts are located and this is what maximizes output.

Compression and pressure can be thought of as complementary pairs. When a muscle is used to create compression, it is creating pressure that the neuromuscular system detects. Without muscular pressure, there is no muscular compression.

The gluteus maximus, on the other hand, in all of its quadrangular glory, is a lever arm. It moves a big bone. And it's shaped and designed in a way to support the movement of that bone.

The muscles that support us and their functions can be summed up like this:

- Compress.
- Apply pressure.
- Create collisions.
- Harness energy.
- Keep it moving.

We will cover some of the other muscles that work as levers in chapters 4 and 5, but remember that muscles work together, not in isolation. One isn't better than the other, and they are all necessary to create and sustain movement.

Torque, another piece of the lever puzzle:

When you turn a hex wrench, is it easier to turn it really close to the screw or is it easier to turn it further away from the screw?

Further away from the screw, right? And that's because of torque, which is a term that refers to angular force. You can apply more rotational force further away from the fulcrum on the lever arm than you can closer to the fulcrum. (Torque is applied on the lever arm. This will become important in a minute.)

Remember from chapter 2 that the fulcrum is also the axis of rotation. When the hex wrench has a long lever arm so that you can turn the hex wrench far away from the axis of rotation, how is the lever arm of the wrench oriented into the screw?

It's perpendicular to the screw (hopefully, this isn't new since we talked about it just a few pages ago).

And what direction do you push the wrench in order for it to begin turning?

Parallel to the axis of rotation.

Again, this isn't new. But it's important, so I am saying it again. Perpendicular and parallel are another complementary pair. Perpendicular refers to the axis of rotation, not to the joint. Joints work in all kinds of positions. What matters is whether the lever arm is compressing into the fulcrum so that there is pressure.

When you push on the wrench, you apply stress to the wrench. Stress can be thought of as any force applied to a structure. It can be internal or external.

The wrench resists the stress you apply, not wanting to change its position.

There is a moment when nothing happens. This is the equivalent of an isometric contraction; the wrench is storing energy. You are storing energy. Neither you or the wrench wants to release your energy.

At some point, you overcome the strength of the wrench. The standoff ends as the wrench relinquishes its energy.

When you overcome the wrench's resistance, it begins turning, changing position. It moves, or deforms.

Stress, strain, and deformation are a threesome we will discuss in more detail in chapter 5, but for now know that in order to move without breaking, there needs to be the right amount of stress and strain. Prior to movement, there will be an isometric contraction that takes place, a resistance of the change of position. Stress–both internal and external–is overcome through internal strength, which produces deformation, a change in shape of the physical structure, or the moment when the hex wrench starts to turn. How long the isometric lasts determines how fast (or slow) the deformation is.

The perpendicular can be compression or expansion. If you reach your arm out to the side so it is perpendicular with your body, there is expansion through the shoulder joint. If you place your hand on the ground with your arm perpendicular to your body there is compression through the shoulder joint.

When your arm is reaching out to the side, you can apply stress to the arm to make it move several different ways. You can move the arm up or down, pushing or pulling. You can move the arm away from midline or towards midline, adducting or abducting. Or you can combine the actions, pushing and adducting, pulling and abducting.

When your hand is on the ground, the same principles apply. If you push the hand away from you, your body will move away from the hand, the arm moving overhead. If you pull the hand towards your body, your body pulls towards your hand. If you pull the hand towards the center of your chest, the body begins to rotate over the hand. If you push the ground in the direction of the pinkie finger, your body will rotate away from your hand. And just like when the hand is reaching out to the side, you can apply a combination of parallel stresses to create a three-dimensional rotation.

Let's get back to the hex wrench. If the hex wrench's lever arm is long and you can easily turn the screw, does the screw turn quickly or slowly?

Kind of slowly, right?

What if the wrench were shorter. Would it be harder or easier to begin turning the screw?

Probably a little bit easier because effort goes a long way for a short lever arm. But would you be able to turn it faster or slower?

Faster, right? That's because short lever arms are strong and allow you to generate speed, but the range will be less (think tighter rotations). A long lever arm gives you range, but at the cost of speed.

Movement exists on a continuum between fast and slow. If a screw isn't very tight, you can use a short hex wrench to remove it very quickly, with minimal effort. Once it gets moving, it moves very fast, like riding a bike with small wheels—your legs spin around at a comical pace and the bike moves forward, seemingly fast. If the screw is tight, a longer hex wrench is the right tool for the job. You can apply more force to generate the rotation needed to unscrew the screw, but the wrench will turn more slowly.

If you got on a bicycle with big wheels and the bike was in a high gear, it would take some effort from your legs to get the wheels turning, but once they started moving, you could sustain the pedal stroke with relatively low effort. The wheels will spin more slowly than if you were riding a small bike, so the speed of rotation is slower. But if the distance from point A to point B is going to take longer than two minutes, you will get there faster on the bike with big wheels.

(Two minutes is a totally arbitrary number. Maybe the actual number is thirty seconds or maybe it's five minutes. Adarian says physics is easy if you don't do the math. I am applying that principle here.)

The same thing happens when you do a flip on a trampoline. If you tuck yourself into a ball to do the flip, less effort is required to initiate the rotation, but the flip will be fast. If instead you keep your body long and fold at your hips into a pike position, more effort will be required to initiate the rotation, but the rotation will be slower. Speed is based on levers, and the function of levers is based on rotation.

The one where you roll over:

Let's say you want to turn over in bed. Is it easier to turn over with your legs extended or with your knees tucked in towards you?

Go ahead and try it. Lie down on your left side. Reach your left legs out and roll over onto your right side.

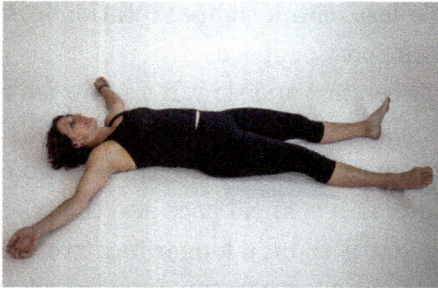

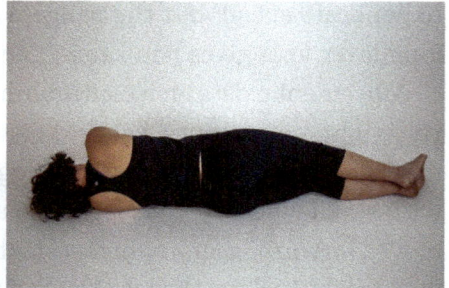

Curl your knees in towards you. Keep your knees curled in as you roll over onto your left side. (If you aren't near a bed, you can perform the same action on the floor.)

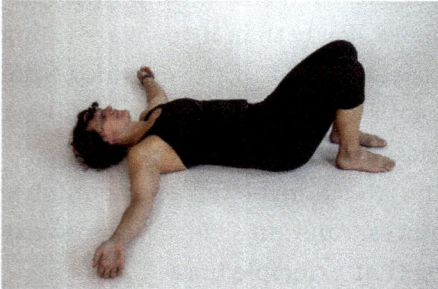

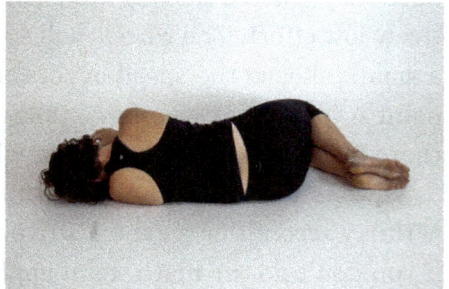

Which variation felt faster? Which variation felt easier?

The faster version is with your knees tucked in towards you.

Why?

Because the lever arm is shorter. When the lever arm is short, you rotate faster. Long lever arm, long rotation, but easier to get going. Short lever arm, short rotation, harder to get going.

Now try this: Perform the same action of rolling over with your knees tucked in, but imagine you are rotating because someone is rolling you over from the left side to the right side at the small of the back. How does that feel?

Now, imagine someone is pushing you over from the right side to the left side at your knees. Which feels easier?

Being pushed from your knees, right? Why?

Because the torque is being applied further away from the fulcrum. This makes the rotation easier.

And, get this (because this is kind of cool). For rotation to occur, the torque would be applied to the place where the thigh is perpendicular to the hip so there is compression. The torque, or the force applied, would be parallel to the hip.

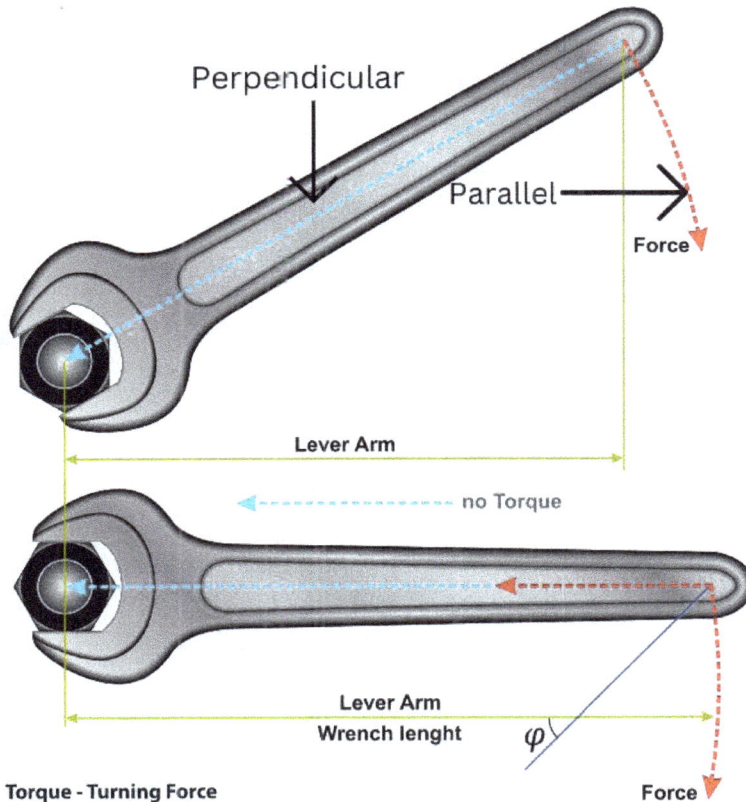

Perpendicular

Parallel

Force

Lever Arm

no Torque

Lever Arm

Wrench lenght

φ

Torque - Turning Force

Force

Remember, compression and pressure are complementary pairs. So are perpendicular and parallel. If you want movement to be efficient, whether that means fast, lingering, strong, or gentle, the complementary pairs matter.

One final note about torque—it requires more torque to get going than it does to keep going.

Go back to the example of rolling over in bed. If someone were to push you over at your knees, they would have to push relatively hard to start the turn, but if you were to roll all of the way over and wanted to keep going, the next time the person pushed you they wouldn't have to push as hard. You would roll more easily, until eventually you were rolling along sideways, unassisted. It takes a lot of torque to get you moving, but very little torque to keep you moving. Speed requires less torque than stillness.

When you initially get on a bike and you push the pedal down, you need to push down a noticeable amount to get the bike moving. Once the bike is moving, you don't have to push down as hard on the pedals. The amount of torque you need is related to the amount of speed you already have—the faster you are going, the less torque is needed. The slower you are going, the more torque is needed.

Put more simply: fast is low input and slow is high input.

Remember the imaginary jar lid you opened earlier? If the jar's lid is tight, what happens?

You have to strain to get the lid to begin twisting. How does this feel?

Hard. You are aware of the pressure of the lid against your hand. You can feel the muscles in your hand working to grip the lid. The amount of input required to produce the desired motor output is high. The corresponding movement of the hand to begin rotating the lid is slow.

What if the jar's lid is loose? What happens when you open the jar?

It twists quickly, easily, without much effort. You barely have time to process the sense of your hand against the lid. The input is low.

Take a moment to think about this from a movement context. If fast is low input and slow is high input, will someone experience more or less sensory input if they are moving fast?

Less. And they will experience more sensory input when they move slow.

If you are starting to feel mildly confused, don't worry. These terms will continue to make more sense as you move through the next few chapters. The main goal is for you to have a basic familiarity with these concepts so when we refer back to them, at least you can go, wait! I read something about that earlier. Familiarity breeds understanding, and understanding is what will enable you to experience a sense of movement mastery

Thinking about movement: The pitch, yaw, roll paradigm shift

At this point, hopefully you understand this body that you possess is composed of several simple tools called levers. Effort is applied to the levers. This creates rotation at a fulcrum point, which creates movement. Movement is a series of rotations, and these rotations can be described through terms that I keep using to describe three-dimensional movement: pitch, yaw, and roll.

When your partner pulls you towards them, how and where they place their hand determines how you move. The movement isn't straight; there's a bit of rotation up, down, sideways, and/or horizontally as you move towards them. How you move towards the person pulling you is a combination of these movements, a multidimensional experience.

As you near your partner, you have a choice. You can resist, applying force back towards them. When you watch two people rolling on a mat doing Brazilian jiujitsu, you see the resistance as one pulls and the other resists in a sort of chess match until someone rotates in a way that allows for an escape.

Martial arts and dance are two examples of interactive disciplines that are based on the successful use of levers in this multidimensional way. It could be argued the success of all movement is based on these concepts, but sometimes we (and by we I mean the people coaching or doing the movements) get fixated on the linear look of the movement, forgetting that the appearance of a linear path is inaccurate.

In traditional movement sciences, movement is often described as an occurrence in the sagittal plane, frontal plane, and transverse plane; movement occurs front to back, side to side, or horizontally.

But when you look at the nuances of movement from a lever perspective, it's happening in a different way; in an oscillatory pattern rather than a straight, linear pattern.

In aviation, flight paths are described using the terms pitch, yaw, and roll. Imagine a kite, traveling through the air. Pitch is what happens when the front of the kite pitches up towards the sky and the back of the kite pitches down towards the earth. The lever arm is the skin of the kite. The fulcrums are the cross sticks that make up the horizontal and vertical axis of the kite. You can think of the fulcrum as the kite's axis of rotation.

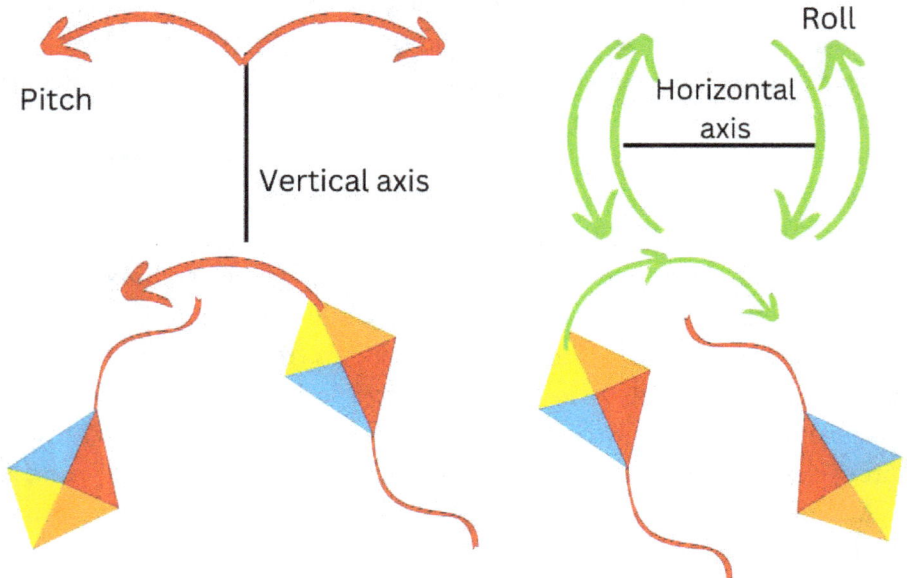

Pitch

Vertical axis

Roll

Horizontal axis

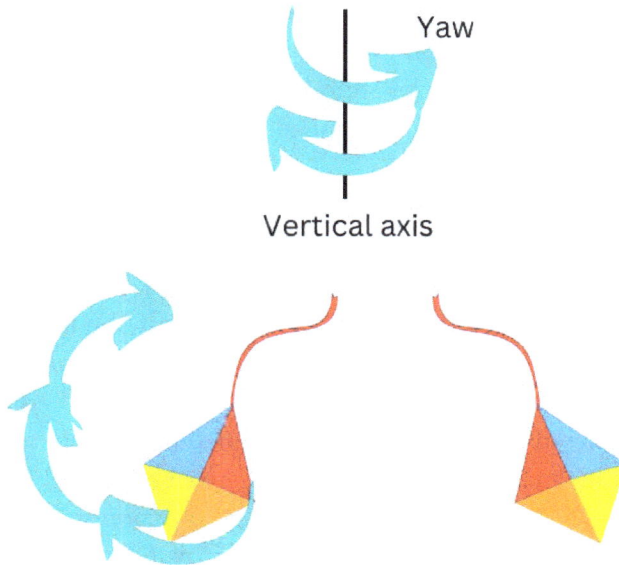

Another way to think of pitch is that it occurs when a box lid open and closes. The lid is the lever arm, the hinge is the fulcrum. The rotation is up and down.

If the front of the kite rotates towards the back of the kite, like a dog looking for its tail, that is yaw. The lever arm is still the body of the kite and the axis of rotation, or fulcrum, is still the center of the kite, but the movement that is occurring there has shifted.

Another way to think of yaw is that it happens when you swing a door left and right. The door hinge is the fulcrum. The door is the lever arm.

Roll occurs when a kite rotates so one side rolls up towards the sky and one side rolls down. The body of the kite is still the lever arm. The fulcrum is still the center of the kite (Ludwig, 2018).

When you take a standard movement like a jumping jack, your arms and legs roll. The lever arms are the arms and legs; the fulcrums are the shoulders and hips.

When you deadlift, you pitch your torso up as you lift the bar. The torso is the lever. The fulcrum is the hips.

When you run, the change of the shin angle pitches you forward. The ankle is the fulcrum point, allowing the foot to both roll and pitch and the shin to pitch forward. The leg may yaw or it may not, depending on how and when the shin angle changes and the rotation occurs around the ankle.

Two people rolling on a mat are producing dynamic, rotational movement. Two people slow dancing are still moving in a rotational way, just more slowly. The lever arms, interestingly, are similar (both forms of movement are anchored in part by the arms), but the intention behind the movements is different. The Brazilian jiujitsu practitioner is trying to impart a collision on another person while limiting the pressure and collisions imparted upon them; the people dancing together are trying to extend the collision and maintain the pressure between them.

When you look at movement that happens at joints, it is (on a very small scale) a combination of pitch, yaw, and roll; when you look at the movement more globally, you will see that it is defined by pitch, yaw, and roll, no matter how it looks initially.

As you move through the next four chapters, you will see the themes of levers and multidimensional movement emerge repeatedly. Don't over-think it, but if you feel yourself getting overwhelmed, step back and ask yourself:

- What is moving?
- What is the lever?
- What is the fulcrum?
- Where is the rotation?
- How is that causing rotation that oscillates out?

And now we move on to the crux of safety, the place where the input can dramatically change the output—the anchor.

CHAPTER 4

ANCHOR YOURSELF TO YOURSELF

You fold in and find an internal sense of connection, one that allows you to connect more intimately with the moment. In order to increase the pressure, you find an anchor point that allows you to compress more deeply to feel the pressure, feel the sensation.

A critical aspect to movement freedom and creating a sense of elation is being able to create a strong anchor. Anchoring is the connection to the ground, a stable external object, or to yourself. There are two types of anchors: necessary and unnecessary.

A necessary anchor enhances movement. For instance, if you are preparing to kick a ball, one foot anchors to allow the other foot to swing freely.

An unnecessary anchor doesn't enhance or detract from movement: it's just blah. If you are standing on one leg while performing a hip circle with the other leg, the standing foot is the necessary anchor. If you hold onto something with your hands while performing the circle, the hands become an unnecessary anchor, not making the movement more coordinated or improving the outcome in any way (though they do, perhaps, stop you from falling over).

If you were to reach out and grab a tree branch on a hike to help you keep your balance and the wood bent under your weight, the branch would be a weak anchor and your ability to remain upright would be challenged.

The tree branch would be an unnecessary anchor, not assisting with the outcome of staying upright.

If the tree branch remained strong, not bending under your weight as you leaned your hand against it, the anchor provided by the branch would be strong. The strength of the anchor would allow you to stay upright and you would feel stable as you plucked your way down the rocky path. The tree branch would become necessary, making you more stable and better able to execute the movement.

An anchor is a reliable source of support; to anchor is to provide a sense of stability to an object or, in this case, the body. In the context of moving, anchoring provides balance to the system, either through compression or through the balance of pressure, a kind of pressurization that gives the body an opportunity to feel connected and secure. The anchor is the green light. It allows the movement to occur.

Compression gives you the ability to rotate. We talked about the hex wrench in chapters 2 and 3, but to recap: in order to actually rotate the wrench, you need to press the head of the wrench into the screw, connecting the wrench and the screw. This creates the anchor. Only then can you apply pressure to the wrench and begin screwing—or unscrewing—the screw. Remember, you need perpendicular to get parallel; you need parallel to begin movement.

Earlier, we talked about muscles that create compression. These can also be thought of as anchoring muscles. The gluteus medius and minimus, for instance, can anchor the femur to the pelvis. This creates compression at the hip joint, which allows the gluteus maximus to rotate the femur behind the body. Without those two muscles, what would happen?

The femur would slip into the joint and there would be no rotation.

Anchoring can occur anywhere you come into contact with something that connects you to the external environment or with yourself. You can anchor yourself to yourself, like when your obliques connect your ribs to your pelvis, or you can anchor yourself to an external object, like when your feet are on the ground or you hold a rigid bar.

Some muscles, like the obliques, can both anchor and rotate. They create compression, which creates pressure. But they also rotate the ribs and spine, which means they can act as a lever arm for the torso.

Imagine you are moving in towards someone, shifting your weight to create more contact. You step your foot closer. You lean your torso in, expecting to make contact with their chest.

Just as you are about to connect, they step back. What happens?

You stumble forward, your feet tumbling forward to catch you. The anchor that you were anticipating would support you isn't there, so your body has to come up with a new anchor to keep you safe and upright.

Anchors shift, depending on the phase of movement you are in and what you are doing. If an anchor disappears, you will find a new way to balance yourself. If an anchor suddenly appears, it will stabilize you, unless, for some reason, you are guarded, you don't trust the anchor, or it is a weak anchor for providing balance.

Imagine you are standing with both feet firmly weighted into the ground. Your gregarious thirty-pound dog comes bounding into you at full speed. What happens?

You might sway a bit, but chances are high you don't actually move or get knocked over because your anchors (the feet) keep you balanced. They are strong. This is different than if your feet were glued into the ground, not allowing any movement to occur. You would tumble, feet rooted and immobile, while the rest of you buckled under the weight of your overly enthusiastic dog.

What if you were kneeling on your legs when your dog came bounding into you? What would happen then?

You would probably fold over, your torso coming close to the ground. Your knees might bend as you tried not to end up one big pile on the floor.

Your knees are a weak anchor, unable to fully support you when your balance is threatened by an outside influence or perturbation. Your feet are a stronger anchor, responding to perturbations through micromovements that allow you to remain upright under a variety of circumstances.

Anchors can be global or local. Global anchors are the main characters, the ones who weigh you down so that the local anchors further up the chain can do their jobs. A strong global anchor influences the work of the local anchors. It's like a good director in a company—when the director is strong, the managers working under the director are positively influenced to do their best work.

Global anchors slow things down. Your foot, when it is transitioning from the air to the ground, becomes a class-one lever. It puts on the brakes so that it can provide the necessary connection to the ground while you move forward.

The local anchors, like the managers, are then free to work in a way that highlights their strengths. Local anchors are things like the obliques or the quadratus lumborum, muscles that anchor the top and bottom halves of the torso that allow the torso to compress and expand. They respond to the stability provided by global anchors of the lower or upper body.

Imagine a baseball player throwing a ball. The global anchors are the feet, which weigh down the rest of the body. The local anchors are the quadratus lumborum and the obliques, which keep the rib cage anchored to the pelvis, providing compression and pressure so that rotation can occur. The rotation of the torso creates rotation in the arm. This allows the arm to be propelled around and forward so the ball can be thrown.

Anchors shift, depending on how you are moving. When you move your shin over your foot, the foot creates a global anchor, acting as the weight that connects you to the ground. When you reach the hand towards something, the obliques become the global anchor, weighing down the upper body; the hand becomes a local anchor as it reaches towards something. Anchors can be either extrinsic or intrinsic, and act to provide a sense of stability and safety for the entire system.

When you anchor yourself to the ground, what is the primary source of connection? Unless you are a professional hand balancer, it's probably your feet. This is convenient, since the feet connect to the lower leg via the ankle and the ankle joint via connective tissue. The connective tissue in the ankle are filled with those specialized cells called mechanoreceptors that I mentioned in chapter 2, which give your brain information about joint position and pressure (Macefield, 2021; Han et al., 2015).

The feet are also filled with those same specialized cells, except instead of being located in the structures around the joint, they are located in the skin. They too detect changes in pressure, but the pressure they sense is the pressure between the skin and the ground rather than the internal pressure that the ankle joint detects (Kennedy & Inglis, 2002).

The ability of the neuromuscular system to get input from the outside landscape and the internal environment is what creates the output. And that input, you will notice, is pressure.

What creates pressure? Compression.

If you are doing a single-leg squat, do you want a lot of input from your neuromuscular system or a little?

What about if you are hiking and you need to leap from one rock to another?

And what happens if you are connecting with someone? Do you want more or less input?

If I am doing a single-leg squat, I want a high degree of input. Otherwise, the balance is going to be challenging, the movement is going to be challenging, and my chances of successfully completing the repetition in a coordinated way (the output), are slim to none.

And where, in this example, is the input coming from? The thing that's in contact with the ground, a.k.a. your anchor—the foot, which is observing ground pressure, and the ankle, which determines how much tension is on it. If there's too much compression at the ankle joint, your ability to successfully perform the squat decreases because too much compression leads to too much pressure—too much pressure leads to sensation.

Since the single-leg squat is a high-input movement, does that make it a movement that is fast or slow?

High-input movements are movements that are slow. Low-input movements are movements that are fast. A single-leg squat is a slow movement.

Before I move on, there are other places that create input as well. The scapula and obliques anchor the top half of the torso to the bottom half. The eyes, ears, and nose take in the input from the external environment, determining whether the system (you) is in a state of homeostasis, meaning internal balance (from chapter 1).

The input all of these areas receive determines the motor output. Or, more simply, the input determines the movement.

Now what about the hiking example? You are preparing to leap from one rock to another. Where is the input coming from?

Similar places, different environments. The hiking shoe is providing input to the foot about the shoe. Your eyes are scanning the environment and determining whether the surface of the rock you are about to leap to is slippery, stable, or somewhere in-between. Conveniently, the foot is still the anchor. This information from the eyes and shoe allows the foot to create flexion at the ankle joint, which is met by the downward pressure of the tibia at the ankle joint. This input determines the output—how and when you leap from one rock to the next.

Is this a low input or a high-input movement?

Low input. In fact, minimizing the amount of time you spend with your foot in contact with the rock will probably make you more successful at maintaining your balance.

In the final example, you are connecting with someone else in a physical way. The anchor is going to come from the other person—are you anchoring your hands against their wrists, or is your body wrapped around theirs? Or maybe your feet are pressing into the surface of the floor as they try and move you. The input also comes from the touch of the other person and the pressure generated by the contact between the two of you. That determines the output, whether the goal is to place the other person in an arm bar, balance on the other person because you are doing AcroYoga, or something more intimate.

Is the connection high input or low input?

High input. Which means the connection is slow, not fast.

The environment determines the anchor:

Imagine you are running in the dark on somewhat rocky terrain. There is no light in the sky because it is a new moon and the stars are covered with clouds. With each step, will your foot land confidently, pressing firmly in the earth to provide a solid connection point? Or will it land carefully, gingerly feeling what's beneath it before it acquiesces to the ground?

For most of us, the above scenario creates a fear of falling, and that fear of falling alters how we move. If you want to move well, you need to feel safe.

This crosses every movement experience. Without a sense of safety, it is difficult to find an anchor. My dad had a serious stroke about seven months ago that left him paralyzed on the left side. Initially, he couldn't even lift his arm up. Because he is a tall man, the ground is far away. Every single time he shifted position or moved, he didn't feel anchored to anything around him. This created a sense of fear.

Fortunately, his clever rehabilitation specialist recognized this, and my dad's girlfriend installed a long bar that was bolted to the floor on the left side of his chair. Now, when he wants to shift positions or stand up, he can anchor both hands to the bar, pressing the bar down as he presses into his feet. This gives him two anchor points, decreasing his sense of instability and increasing his sense of safety.

One way to create a sense of safety is to do what the rehabilitation specialist did for my dad—create an anchor. Your anchor will give your neuromuscular system the feedback that it craves, allowing you to produce efficient movement, movement that can be fast and forceful, slow and sensual, and everything in between.

When you perform repetitions of something like a single-leg squat, you set up the movement (input) and do the movement (output). The outcome (whether or not you successfully performed the single-leg squat) determines if you use the same set up for the next repetition. The environment is presumably safe. You have plenty of room, minimal distractions, and minimal extra-sensory input.

When you are hiking and you come to a place where you need to leap from one rock to another, your set up is influenced by your previous experience and whatever sensory input you are getting from your other senses. Are you able to simply react, leaping from rock- to-rock without thinking about it? Or do you have to think about how you are going to leap from rock to rock? One of these generally leads to a better outcome than the other.

When you are connecting physically with someone, you are assessing the intent of the other person. Are they acting in a tender way or a harmful way? This information is determined by your senses and based on previous experience with the individual. The output is based on whether there is a sense of trust or distrust—do you lean into the person or push them away?

Creating internal safety: Compression, pressure, and anchoring

Creating a sense of safety comes from making smart choices about your environment and where you are training, but you can also create this internal sense of safety through terms you are (hopefully) already pretty familiar with: using the right amount of compression to create the desired amount of pressure so you can add weight to your anchor.

This concept can be utilized anywhere movement takes place. Where does movement take place in the human body? At joints. And joints, it turns out, love having feedback that makes them feel safe. In the absence of balanced pressure and compression (input), a number of things happen, including less efficient use of the lever (the brain will bypass the range of motion that it deems unsafe), and/or sensation in the form of...well, sensation.

Sensation means lots of things. Sometimes it means the sense of discomfort. Sometimes it means the sense of tightness or instability. Sensation indicates the brain is perceiving something is off. Whether that something is an actual injury or is inadequate input leading to less-than-optimal output is up to a medical professional to decide.

Too little or too much pressure leads to too little or too much compression. When you understand levers, anchors, and pressure, you can dial things up or down until you find just the right balance point between sensing and sensation.

Where the earth meets the body:

You press through your feet, arching your back up, feeling a deep connection resonate through you. As you reach through your feet a little bit more, your pelvis responds, tilting.

Your feet are your source of connection to the ground. They allow you to create movement through the pelvis and hips (just like the pelvis and hips can allow you to create movement through the feet). The feet can only act as a strong lever when they are on the ground, operating as a class-one or class-two lever, depending on whether they are slowing you down or speeding you up. (Please see appendix for the full break down.) It should make sense that one of the most impactful places to create a feeling of safety for your entire neuromuscular system is through the joints of the feet; the feet and ankles are rich with sensory input.

When I originally wrote the above paragraph, I wrote that the feet allow you to create movement. Adarian corrected me, "You are the movement. And what are you trying to do? You are trying to move the ground. And by trying to move the ground, you move."

It's worthwhile to remember that the origin of all movement is within you, a response by your brain and spinal cord based on the input received.

When input creates stress, you respond with strain to prevent the stress. The result is a shift of your body, a movement of some kind.

We are going to look at the joints of the foot through the context of anchoring, compression, pressure, and as a fulcrum, but keep in mind that the sensory information coming from the ankle and foot contribute significantly to your ability to create an anchor. The anchor creates the balance. Balance is an output that is the result of the input we talked about earlier. Proprioception, along with the input from your inner ear and eyes, keep you standing (Bronstein, 2016). As Adarian said, "downstream controls everything upstream." The feet are downstream.

One of the things I learned while writing this book is that the concepts discussed on these pages can be seen in the way researchers test aspects of movement. For instance, one way researchers test how much proprioception contributes to your ability to remain upright is to vibrate the Achilles tendon. We talked about vibrations in chapter 1, but to recap: movement creates collisions. Collisions create vibrations. Vibrations are either wanted or unwanted. Unwanted vibrations are dealt with by throwing you off-balance or altering a movement pattern.

The vibrations provided by the researchers are unwanted. They aren't backed up by anything else that is meaningful to the neuromuscular system, like impact or movement. The result? Subjects sway backwards as their central nervous systems try to figure out how to deal with an undesired input, an input that affects the ability to anchor through the feet (Eysel-Gosepath et al., 2016).

Think of things that throw you off-balance: curbs, rocks, ice, cars, people. Even the air (unless I am the only one who has been walking along, totally not in the present moment because I am pondering nothing particularly interesting, only to find myself stumbling over nothing).

What happens when your balance gets knocked off? You either catch yourself (sometimes miraculously) with your feet landing underneath you or you end up on the ground, dazed, unsure what just happened.

Neither situation feels particularly great. You might feel jarred or like you jammed your foot into the ground to catch you. Like the boxer from chapter 1, stumbling causes you to be the recipient of an uncontrolled collision, leading to unwanted vibrations.

If you have good input from the foot, the collisions you deal with during your everyday life will be more controlled. Think of what happens when you roll over your foot as you walk. The pressure in the foot shifts from where your foot hits the ground to the forefoot (front of the foot) (Wu et al., 2020). How this occurs is based on the structure of the foot, the surface of the ground, whether you're wearing platforms or running shoes, and a myriad of other factors.

This also means the heel doesn't spend that much time on the ground while you are moving because as the shin angle changes, the contact with the foot against the ground changes. Imagine a narrow squat: if I squat all of the way down to my heels, my shin angle is going to shift forward. In order to create the perpendicular needed for ankle flexion, my heels will lift slightly off the floor. If my heels remain on the floor, what happens?

I am no longer creating balanced pressure in the ankle joints. My shinbones can't apply pressure perpendicularly because the feet are no longer in a position that allows that to happen. This alters my ability to use the feet as an anchor and my ankles as a fulcrum.

When you look at people across a wide variety of sports and athletics, you will begin to notice a common position from which they initiate movement. This position, slightly squatted, butt down, heels slightly up, head free to scan the environment, is also commonly used by runners and is commonly known as "sitting in the bucket."

In the running world, sitting in the bucket is considered bad, as though running slightly squatted is going to somehow ruin any chances you have of moving quickly. It's frequently cited as a source of injury, except there is no research to back up this statement, just like there is no research that suggests sitting in the bucket is inefficient or leads to slow times.

In fact, sitting in the bucket can be seen in some of the fastest people in the world. Eliud Kipchoge. Almaz Ayana. Joshua Cheptegei. Letesenbet Gidey. All world record holders as of this writing. All people who sit in the bucket.

Sitting in the bucket creates a solid anchor, an anchor that allows the ground to move underneath you as the body shifts forward. This anchor sets up everything else: pressure, compression, levers, and controlling collisions. Remember, downstream controls upstream. Sitting in the bucket sets up downstream. Everything else follows.

As Adarian says, "to move well you have to sit in the bucket." It doesn't matter whether you are a tennis player, runner, or martial artist; sitting in the bucket sets the foundation for moving well.

Sitting in the bucket and squats:

Sitting in the bucket anchors the entire body as one. We mentioned a moment ago that sitting in the bucket is a squatted position, but do squats in the gym resemble sitting in the bucket on the court or the track?

No. In fact, squats in the gym have a lot of rules you are "supposed" to follow. These rules are designed to create a certain shape that helps you lift a lot of weight.

Putting your heels down is commonly instructed during squats, all kinds of squats, regardless of foot position or whether it's a two-legged squat or a single-legged squat. And what happens if someone can't keep their heels down? They are given ankle mobility drills to improve their ability to keep their heels down.

Are ankle mobility drills the best choice to create an effective anchor and an effective fulcrum?

No. When the heel comes off the ground, the surface area between your foot and the ground is decreased. This increases pressure and reduces the amount of compression needed to create an anchor.

Put more simply, smaller surface areas require less compression to create a secure anchor. And secure anchors allow for fluid movement.

Remember what happens with a lot of compression?

A lot of pressure.

And what happens when there's too much pressure?

Sensation.

Ankle flexion and arches: The untold story

People often confuse the term ankle pronation with a falling transverse arch or pronation at the forefoot (a downward rotation of the front of the foot towards the ground). For the purposes of this book, we are eliminating any references to pronation. Instead, here and forevermore, we will refer to the movement that occurs at the front of the ankle joint as ankle flexion. This is the movement that allows the foot to rotate towards the ground while maintaining integrity of the arch, allowing arches to do what they do: withstand compression. Ankle flexion is a combination of the three-dimensional movement terms we discussed in chapter 3: pitch, yaw, and roll.

When the foot creates an anchor during upright movement, the ankle becomes a fulcrum. The ankle joint can be thought of as the meeting place of three different bones: the talus, tibia, and fibula (the tibia and fibula are your shinbones). The ankle joint is bordered by two bones that jut out on the inside and outside of your ankle (Manganaro & Alsayouri, 2022).

During an activity like running, there is the briefest moment where the foot acts like a brake. "The anchor allows the brake to work," Adarian explained. "It does this through increasing pressure and reducing surface area." This ensures that when the parallel action is applied by the hip to create the rotation of the leg (remember back to levers and rotation in chapters 2 and 3), the fulcrum at the ankle doesn't slip. The braking action is a critical piece in allowing the body to move forward.

Pressure creates input. Compression creates pressure. So the compression of the shinbone down into the ankle allows for rotational movement to occur.

Try this: come into a tall half-kneeling position with your right foot forward. Place your hands on the top of the right shinbone near your knee. Run your hands down the front of the shinbone, generating downward pressure with your hands, into your shin, into your ankle. Do this three times. Each time you run your hands down along the shinbone, imagine the shinbone is rooting down into the center of the ankle joint.

After your third one, stand up. Imagine the action of the right shinbone rooting down into the ankle as you bend your right knee and straight it a few times. You might even try stepping your left foot forward and back as you continue to focus on the right shinbone reaching down into the ankle.

When you finish, pause. Does your right leg feel different than your left leg?

What just happened? You created pressure at the right ankle joint. This sent feedback up into the brain and created a clearer map of the area, which your brain can then (hopefully) take into account the next time you move. It's a beautiful system when you give it space, and the right input, to create efficient movement.

Now that pressure and, in turn, compression, have been created, rotation can occur. Here's where things get really interesting: there is rotation that occurs at the ankle joint and rotation that occurs over the ankle joint. The ankle moves into ankle flexion while the shin rotates up and over the ankle (depending on what you're doing).

Oy, that's even dizzying to write out, so let's make it less complicated. Ankle rotates one way. Shin rotates another. Movement looks like it's occurring because everything is moving forward, when really it's a series of rotations.

Ankle flexion happens after there has been compression at the joint from the shinbone. The ankle then rotates down and towards the ground, bringing the medial malleolus (big bone on the inside of the ankle joint), towards the ground.

People often confuse lateral ankle flexion with the arches collapsing, which it isn't. The arches are kind of amazing and are designed to deal with the compressive forces that occur whenever the feet are on the ground by pushing the compressive forces along the curve of the arch towards the ends of the arch. This makes tension in the arch negligible ("Building Bridges," 2017).

This means the arches don't collapse as the ankle flexes. They receive the compression from the movement, maintaining their shape. It's an incredible design, one that has worked for literally thousands of years to enable us to walk, run, leap, and jump.

Let's talk about arches, baby:

I keep mentioning the foot and its structure, and now I am talking about arches, so let's clarify these mysterious arches and how they allow you to distribute pressure across a relatively small surface area.

For the purposes of this section we are going to consider five arches of the foot. Three of the arches are longitudinal. This means they run lengthwise along the inside and outside of the foot. The fourth arch is transverse, which means it runs horizontally across the ball of the foot, and the fifth arch runs in-line with the big toe.

The medial longitudinal arch runs from the center of the heel to the big toe ball of the foot. If you are reading this while sitting down, pick up your left foot, rest it on your right knee, and run your right fingers from the center of the left heel to the big toe ball of the foot. You will likely feel the natural arch that occurs (Little, 2022).

The arch is supported by the shape of the bones, ligaments, and muscles. Remember that arches resist compression, so this arch doesn't collapse when you place weight on it. Instead, it disperses the load along its length.

The lateral longitudinal arch runs from the center of the heel to the ball of the pinky toe. You can feel it by running your fingers from the center of the heel to the pinky toe ball of the foot. How does this arch compare to the medial longitudinal arch?

While you can probably still feel the formation of an arch, it's flatter than the arch on the inside of the foot.

When you shift your weight into one foot, the lateral longitudinal arch stiffens to support the weight of the body. When it is fully formed, the outer edge of the foot will be long, in contact with the ground until the heel begins to lift.

How does the shape of the foot in the picture resemble the arch of the bridge? Can you see the shape of the arch on both the inside and the outside edge of the foot?

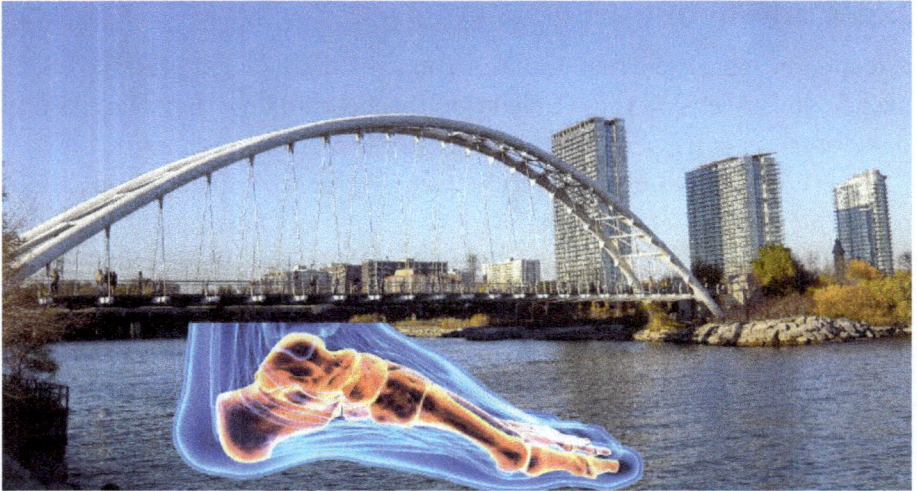

This arch is also supported by bones, ligaments, and muscles. Additionally, the plantar aponeurosis, a sheet of tissue on the bottom of the foot, also acts to support the shape of the arch.

If the lateral longitudinal arch isn't in contact with the floor when the foot is on the ground, what do you think that means for its ability to disperse load across the arch?

It's probably not going to be able to disperse load very well since the arch won't be fully formed. In the exercise section, you will learn how to create a lateral longitudinal arch so that you can take advantage of this aspect of the foot (see exercise 8).

If you look at the outside of your foot you will notice something interesting about the metatarsal bone of the pinky toe. It curves, creating a third arch on the outside of the foot that runs from approximately the middle of the outside edge of the foot to the pinky toe ball of the foot. This arch is different from the other arches because it is a single bone, suggesting the outside edge of the foot is important for distributing pressure.

The fourth arch is the transverse arch. It runs along the ball of the foot, connecting the lateral longitudinal arch and the medial longitudinal arch. You can feel it by running your fingers along the ball of the foot.

It's shorter than the other two, but you will still feel the gentle arch that forms.

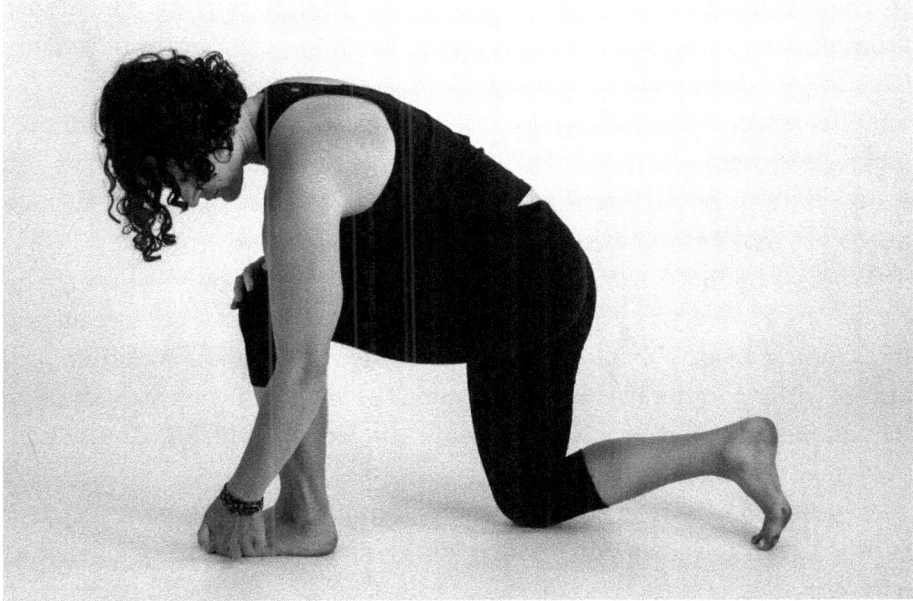

Like the lateral longitudinal arch, the transverse arch is supported by bones, ligaments, muscles, and the plantar aponeurosis. The transverse arch is responsible for up to 40% of the longitudinal stiffness of the foot (Venkadesan et al., 2020). This means that if you want to maximize the spring in your step and have a foot that's working well, you need all of these arches to work together. How can you make that happen?

Since the transverse arch is the meeting point for the longitudinal arches, both of the longitudinal arches need to act as strong arches for the transverse arch to be strong and provide stiffness to the structure of the foot.

The fifth arch is on the outside edge of the big toe. It's a notch alongside the big toe that is made up of the bone. As the foot pitches down while you run, the foot rotates around this point, allowing you to rotate and flex at the same time. This gives you the space to move forward. So you aren't actually pushing the big toe into the ground while you run; you are rotating over it. This rotation allows you to move forward.

How do you create strong arches? Through body mapping. The arches are there. Everyone has them. Tapping into them is a matter of sensing because sensing is input. And input is output.

When do you use your arches? When the foot is on the ground, preparing to propel you forward. Or to the side. Or up in the air. Or if you rotate your body 180 degrees. The arches of the foot create the stiffness needed to move you quickly from one place to another.

When your foot leaves the ground, it no longer needs to be stiff. The arches aren't necessary, just like they aren't necessary if you are sitting or standing around drinking a glass of wine at a friend's wedding. The arches withstand the stress of gravity and the weight of your body through load dispersion and function to create the axis of rotation from which movement occurs.

Try this: Come into a tall half-kneeling position with your left foot forward. Tap the inside anklebone with your fingers, getting a sense of where that is.

Place your hands under your left kneecap in the front of the shin. Reach the left pinky toe out. Imagine the outside edge of the left foot is long.

Use your hands to press the shinbone done into the ankle. As you do that, let the ankle respond by feeling how it rotates down and towards the floor. You can even take one hand to the inside anklebone so that when you press the shin down, you can use the hand to gently press the inside anklebone down. Do this three or four times.

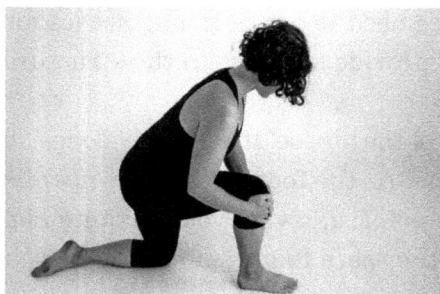

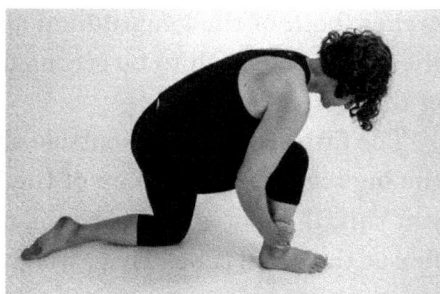

Once you understand the feeling of flexion, see if you can feel your ankle flexion during basic movements like squats and lunges. If you can't feel the action of ankle flexion, ask yourself if you are allowing the shinbone to move down and/or if the pinky toe is continuing to reach out and the outside edge of the foot is long.

What about how the shinbone moves over the ankle? How does that work?

Come back into the tall half-kneeling position with your left foot forward. Place your hands under the left kneecap. Root the shinbone down. Allow the shin *to rotate forward* over the ankle. This part is important. If you think of the shin rotating forward rather than moving forward, your relationship with the movement will be different. How? Because of what happens in the foot.

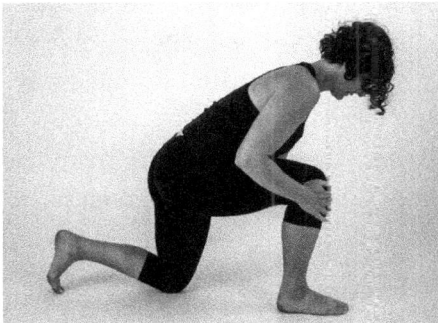

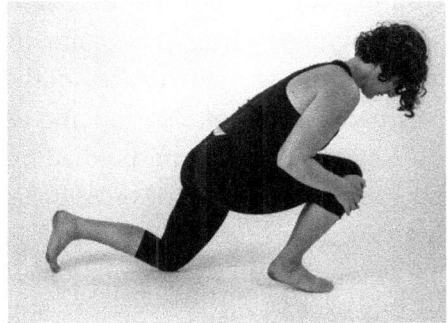

When the shin rotates over the foot versus moving over the foot, the heel won't stay fixed on the ground. At some point, it will lift up. Your foot remains the anchor point despite this new arrangement and is allowed to operate in a more efficient position as a class-one lever versus a class-two lever (see appendix for a quick review on the three different types of levers).

When the shin moves forward over the foot rather than rotates, it's easier to keep the heel on the ground. While this can have its advantages, if you are trying to move forward in space because you are walking or running, you want a coordinated movement between the shin and foot. The result of this coordinated movement? The weight transferring through the foot and the heel lifting, not staying on the ground.

When you change timing and sequencing of a movement because of how you are doing the movement, you affect strength and speed.

Think about this for a moment: if you want to take up running and you are training yourself to keep the heel of the foot on the ground as long as possible in movements like single-leg squats and lunges, does that positive carry over to running?

Probably not. (And to be clear, single-leg squats and lunges don't have a whole lot of transfer to running, but sometimes when you focus on one element in skills that you are training, like keeping the heel down, that intention transfers to other movement patterns, like running.)

When a heel lingers on the ground a beat too long in a movement like running, the anchor is prevented from switching smoothly. Because that's what happens when you are moving dynamically—the anchors smoothly switch, from one location to another as your body continually finds ways to create a sense of internal and external connection.

When you are being pushed on a swing, the anchor shifts from the person pushing you, to you and the swing, then back to the person pushing you. There is a fluidity to it, a back-and-forth, giving and receiving between you and the person pushing.

If one of you is off, the dynamic interplay is no longer fluid. When I used this example back in chapter 1, it was to illustrate unwanted vibrations. Those unwanted vibrations occur, in part, because the anchors aren't being allowed to shift in a way that is in rhythm, harmonious to the natural shift of support from one person to the other.

The anchors can go from global to local anchors internally. When you run and both feet are off the ground, the anchor shifts to the torso so that you can anchor to yourself since nothing else is anchoring you to the world. When your foot lands the anchor shifts back to the foot as the cycle begins again.

We will continue to explore how the ability to shift anchors allows for continuous motion in the next chapters.

CHAPTER 5

PAIRS AND THREESOMES

You allow the vibrations to echo through you, guiding the collisions so you can control their force. The vibrations from their impact reverberate, guiding you to the next movement, allowing you to maintain connection and enabling you to control the input so that the output is what you desire.

To truly experience elation during movement, there needs to be an element of give-and-take, just like when imaginary you was being pushed on a swing last chapter. This give-and-take requires the complementary pairs we have touched upon to exist in an uninterrupted way. When this occurs, movement is unlocked and you are able to freely rotate, spin, and fall with control. These movements, also known as pitch, yaw, and roll, can occur quickly, slowly, or somewhere in-between, depending on the needs of the moment.

This give-and-take is what allows anchors to shift fluidly. When the give-and-take is happening in a way that is complementary, the foot can go from slowing things down to speeding things up. The anchors can shift, from one foot to another, or from the foot to the torso, or from the foot to the hand.

Complementary pairs: A review

You feel an electrical spark as your hands connect. The movement that follows is easy, almost as though you are perfectly in sync, balancing the pressure of each other as you shift. You are the perfect complement to each other as you dance, communicating solely through your touch.

Before we explore pitch, yaw, and roll, let's review complementary and adversarial pairs: what they are and why they matter, along with some examples.

Complementary pairs are two things that enhance the qualities of each other. They work well by themselves, but together they make amazing things happen. Peanut butter and jelly. Coffee and cream. Superman and Lois Lane. "Complementary pairs work better together than apart," Adarian explained when we were talking about it. While they are capable of success solo, they work better together.

A good example of this is a 1D movement versus a 2D movement. A 1D movement would be something like lifting the heel off of the ground. The heel pitches up for this to happen, and while this is a totally fine movement, when the foot also rolls as the heel pitches up, the connection with the foot against the floor becomes more powerful. The complementary pair of pitch and roll creates a 2D movement that will make the foot a more effective lever than just pitch by itself.

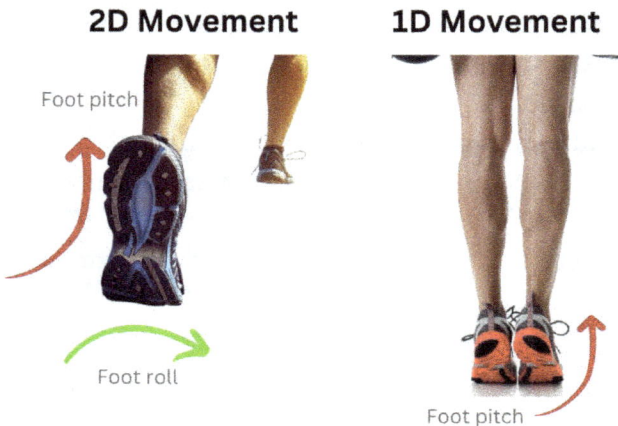

2D Movement

Foot pitch

Foot roll

1D Movement

Foot pitch

Adversarial pairs: The counterpart

Adversarial pairs are two things that are in conflict with each other when they are apart, but are strong when they work together. Breakfast for dinner. Black and white. Yin and yang. Masculine and feminine. Controlled chaos.

When you place adversarial pairs together, the forces are initially in opposition. But upon closer inspection, you see that they actually weave together to create something interconnected. That interconnectedness creates something that is strong when they are balanced just right. Adversarial pairs depend on homeostasis; without homeostasis, the feminine can overwhelm the masculine or the black can mute the white.

When you move, adversarial pairs create the isometric contraction. They oppose one another, creating an optimal amount of stress and strain for the desired action so you can be stable or rotate, moving through the world with an element of control.

Complementary pairs and adversarial pairs maintain balance. They create an environment where homeostasis becomes a baseline that is easily returned to, rather than something that the system seeks. When homeostasis is the rule rather than the exception, magic happens.

Sometimes, two things can be complementary pairs initially, only for the relationship to turn toxic when one aspect of the pair becomes more than the other can handle. Think of a standard training concept like volume and strength. How do tissues get stronger? By applying regular stress to the system in the form of work. How do tissues get injured? By applying too much stress to the system in the form of work.

How do tissues get weaker? By applying not enough stress to the system in the form of work.

So whether volume and strength (or work and strength) are complementary is context dependent. When it comes to movement, creating the optimal context is key for creating optimal performance.

Let's review some complementary and adversarial pairs that we have already discussed throughout the previous chapters.

Compression and expansion, a complementary pair:

Compression is the reduction of volume. It is a movement inward, folding towards something. It creates the pressure needed to feel safe.

It also slows things down—when you exhale, your organs compress slowly so that they don't crash into each other.

Whenever you move, you need to create space so that you can move into space. Compression happens when you move into that space. If you move into it in a chaotic way, the resulting collision is jarring. As you dance with someone else, when you move into the space they create for you, you slow down. When you throw a ball at a high speed, as the arm releases the ball, it slows down to move into the space created for it by the leg and torso. Otherwise, it would crash forward, sending strong, undesired vibrations up the arm. Compression is the body's natural braking system, a way to control the impact that occurs from the act of moving.

Expansion is when something increases in size or volume. Expansion relieves the system of pressure as you create space to move into, speeding up movement. When you inhale, the lungs and diaphragm increase in size, expanding to create compression in the abdominal cavity. The response is a decrease in pressure in the intra-abdominal cavity. The stress from the strain of the compression of the rib cage encourages you to inhale more.

This decrease in pressure creates more space into which the organs can move.

This means every time you complete a breath cycle, there is compression and expansion. This cycle allows internal movement whenever you breathe.

When you dance with your partner, you create space for them by expanding so they can move closer, moving quickly so that you don't collide. If you both expand away, the space between you will seem large, a chasm that can appear difficult to fill until one of you begins to move into it, occupying the space that was originally empty.

When you wind up to throw a ball, you pick up speed as you expand your torso back, creating an opening for your body and arm to fall into as you release the ball. If you don't create the space to throw into, when you release the ball it will land near your feet, unable to travel far because you—and thus, the ball— had nowhere to go.

Expanding is when you take the brakes off, creating an opportunity, an unfilled space for possibility.

Movement is a dynamic interplay between compression and expansion. Without one, movement becomes stilted, less fluid, and less efficient. The complement lies in the back-and-forth between the two.

Remember that muscles that cross joints either create compression or expansion. They slow things down or speed things up based on input.

Compression and compression, an adversarial pair:

Imagine a basketball player who excels at dribbling low. They can navigate easily around the feet of the other players and understand how to keep the ball near to the ground. They are very comfortable with navigating the court with the ball in hand.

Compressing through the torso and the legs, which the basketball player is doing when they stay low, allows the player to receive more input from the joints and makes the levers more efficient. This means that when the player needs to jump up to pass the ball or shoot, the ball easily becomes an extension of the arm and the player can rapidly change positions with control.

This is actually an amazing thing—the ability to control the collision improves when there is a high amount of input. A lot of input allows the collision to be controlled automatically, without effort.

When you step off a curb, the input you get from the foot right before it leaves the curb sets you up for success so you don't crash into the ground. Some of the muscles facilitate the lengthening of the foot stepping down. Others allow the anchored leg to stay low, supporting you while you shift the weight over and towards the leg that's stepping, and others anchor the limbs to the body, providing compression as the feet navigate from a higher position to a lower position (Hody et al., 2019). How and when the muscles contract to navigate the stepping down task depends on how the levers are set up—this determines the input, which determines the output (Hagen & Valero-Cuevas, 2017).

Expansion and expansion, another adversarial pair:

Imagine you are running and you vault over a log, the left hand on the log and the right foot on the log. As the left foot prepares to leave the ground to move through the space created by the hand, body, and foot, what needs to happen?

That's actually a trick question because lots of things need to happen, but let's focus on the muscle that connects the pelvis to the back of the knee. It expands the hip and the knee at the same time, allowing the leg to straighten and move back before it swings up and over the log.

The long head of the biceps femoris, a fancy anatomy word referring to part of the hamstring muscle, is a biarticular muscle. This means it crosses two joints; a muscle that crosses two joints plays an important role in how levers are used (Kohei et al., 2021).

We talked about biarticular muscles in chapter 3, but to recap: biarticular muscles allow rotation to happen. Rotation comes from a combination of pitch, yaw, or roll. If there is just pitch, the movement is considered a 1D movement. If there is pitch and yaw or pitch and roll, the movement becomes 2D.

For example, if you reach your leg straight out in front of you with no bend in the knee and the foot pointing straight ahead, the leg would be pitching up. If you reach your leg straight out in front of you and the foot rotates out, the leg would be pitching and yawing.

What allows the leg to reach forward without rotating? Muscles that flex the hip.

What allows the leg to reach forward and the foot to rotate out? The muscles that both flex the hip and extend the knee.

What prevents any twisting from occurring at the knee when you place your straight leg on the ground?

The biarticular muscles. They are create an isometric contraction, preventing too much twisting from happening at the knee joint. (Twisting refers to the shin rotating one way while the thigh rotates the other.)

When the knee is extending and the hip is extending, the hamstring muscle is expanding at the hip and at the knee. Expansion and expansion are adversarial pairs—when they are combined in just the right amount, they neutralize the collision from the ground; the collision provides the necessary input to propel the leg up and over the log. Too much expansion in both areas would cause conflict, slowing the leg to a halt so instead of neutralizing the collision, the collision would vibrate throughout the muscle.

One of the unique properties of biarticular muscles is that they can act in a variety of combinations of expansion and compression, depending on how you are using that specific limb as a lever (in this case, the upper leg). The implications of all of these different combinations means they play a large role in providing sensory input, which affect motor output.

Expansion and expansion is also what allows a shot-putter to release the shot put so it flies through the air. As the throwing arm extends, preparing to release the shot put, the shoulder blade expands across the back. The expansion translates all of the way to the shot put, which can then fly forward in space.

What happens if there's too much expansion? If you brace your torso with the lungs fully inflated and you try to take an inhale, there's no space left for the inhale. The feeling that follows is one of constriction—the expansion becomes compression.

Remember: adversarial pairs work together when there is an element of balance. When that balance is tipped, instead of the adversarial pair facilitating a more effective outcome, the adversarial pair becomes more like Eminem and Rihanna in the song, "Love the Way You Lie"— they start off as the perfect complement, until the house is being burned down.

Compression and collision, a complementary pair:

Compressions and collisions are complementary pairs. The compression slows down the collision until the collision eventually wins. When you collide into something, "the collision generated by compression," Adarian said, "tempers the collision. If not, you're jacked."

Imagine a javelin thrower as they release the javelin. The torso is compressed and rotated, allowing the javelin to fly through the air. The collision generated by the throw forces the javelin thrower to take a step forward, as though they are falling. The impact from the fall forward is reduced by the compression of the torso.

When you compress, energy is redirected away from you. When energy isn't redirected through compression generated by you, the compression is generated by gravity.

What happens when gravity becomes the generator of compression?

The collision isn't controlled, which means the energy isn't redirected in a controlled way. Space isn't created for you to move into and unwanted vibrations echo throughout the body.

Compression happens when a boxer takes a punch or you lay your partner down in bed. If the boxer expands versus compressing, impact feels much greater than rolling with the punch. If your partner tries to extend out as you set them down, they will feel heavy, and the impact will seem jarring.

While compression allows the boxer to roll with the punch and feel less impact, it sets them up to be knocked off-balance. So compression can create vulnerability, depending on the context.

Even an activity like running depends on compression of the foot. When compression and collision are a complementary pair, it looks like this:

- The foot hits the ground.
- The ground pushes up.
- The foot pushes back down.

- A standoff ensues because both the foot and the ground are trying to take up the same space (compression and collision).
- The ankle flexes and gets out of the way, acting as a neutralizer so the weight can shift forward. The heel rises up.

When there isn't compression and collision, it looks like this:

- The foot hits the ground.
- The foot tries to pull up from the ground but it can't, because the weight hasn't moved forward yet.
- The ankle doesn't get out of the way. The foot and ground try to take up the same space, but this time the foot has nowhere to go because no space has been created by the ankle.

In this situation, there is no compression at the foot, preventing it from moving into a class-two lever and allowing the heel to lift.

What does this look like when you run? If the heel stays on the ground as the body passes over it, the ankle probably isn't flexing and the foot isn't moving into a class-two lever. This is kind of like running flat footed.

If the heel lifts as the body passes over the foot, the ankle is more than likely flexing and the foot is moving from a class-one to a class-two lever.

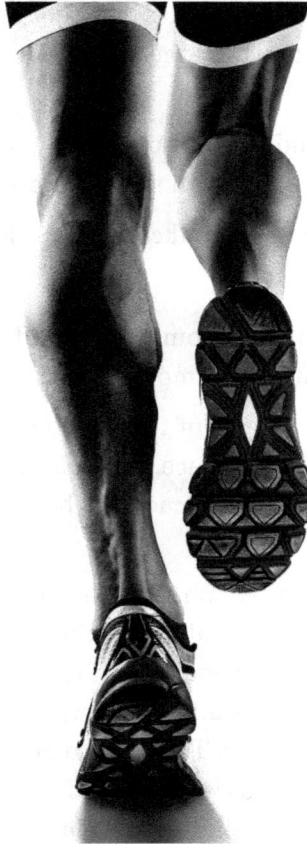

When you run, the hip wants to move up; the shoulder blade compresses to push the hip down. This compression/compression is what allows you to control the impending collision from the ground. What would it look like if the shoulder blade didn't compress down to compress the hip down?

If you are old enough to remember the show *Friends*, there is an episode where the character Phoebe goes for a run with Rachel. "Guys, I'm telling you, when she runs she looks like a cross between Kermit the Frog and the Six Million Dollar Man," Rachel tells everyone later. Phoebe's running style is an exaggerated example of what it looks like when there is no compression (and maybe no basic coordination, either).

Collisions and levers, a complementary pair:

There is a moment of impact with every move that you make. You collide with the wall you are punching. You collide with the ground as you step. You collide with the hand you want to hold.

These collisions are controlled by you, and since you are a collection of simple machines called levers, then really, the collisions are controlled by levers. How you control the impact determines what happens next, and the levers you use are determined by input.

Every collision that is dynamic requires a lever. The efficiency of the lever is what determines how well you collide with the world around you, which is important since the collision creates vibration.

Input and output, a complementary pair:

When you are developing in utero, you spontaneously move (researchers call this "motor babbling"). This allows you to explore your space, and is unrelated to sensation (Fagard et al., 2018).

As you develop in utero, this spontaneous movement begins allowing you to map your body. Interestingly, fetuses like touching the parts of themselves that are sensation rich—the thumb is filled with sensory information. So is the tongue, which is one of the reasons thumb-sucking might be such a common activity during development in the womb. The feet and the eyelids are filled with mechanoreceptors, so it's not surprising you probably spent time touching and rubbing both of those areas while you were gestating.

Because you were rewarded with sensation, certain movements (thumb-sucking, foot rubbing), were repeated. The output provided the input. The input was the chemicals you were rewarded with that flooded your system, encouraging you to repeat the behavior. The input prompted a recurrence of the output.

Once you are out of the womb and are a fully developed adult, the input you receive from those body parts and from the world around you determines how you move. When you change the input, the output changes. Input can change voluntarily, through training certain patterns or behaviors, or involuntarily. If you lose a limb or suffer a brain injury, input changes, so output changes (Makin et al., 2020).

The input, which is both conscious and unconscious, is the key to the output. The output can be thought of as your response. The response determines how you navigate—and experience—the world around you.

Input and output, an adversarial pair:

Input and output can also become adversarial. When two people fighting realize they have a connection, the fighting becomes less rough, more gentle, and turns into something else. The input from the environment, both internal and external, alters the output in subtle ways until the entire intention shifts.

The opposite can also be true. If the input you are receiving indicates danger, the output is modified to protect you. If I am climbing up a pole with the intention to hook my leg around it and lean back without hands but the surface is wet when I hook my leg, I will grasp the pole tighter with both my legs and hands. This will happen fast, without any conscious awareness on my part as my nervous system prioritizes safety over intention. The input overrides the intended output.

A brief note about input, output, and training:

As you rock your pelvis, the muscles around it shift position, creating a change in pressure. Your shin moves forward. Your thigh responds, creating yet another shift throughout the pelvis. You finish by rotating your shoulder blade, altering the position of the muscles that connect the very bottom of the ribs and lumbar spine to the pelvis.

This action can be performed quickly, with the goal of moving through space as fast as possible. You don't have time to sense or feel. The input is low.

Or it can be performed slowly, sensually, as you feel all of the different pieces and how they connect. You purposefully hover in the sensation. The input you receive is high.

Low input means there isn't a lot of extra stuff to contend with. Extra stuff can mean a lot of things. A heavy weight would qualify as extra stuff. So does moving slowly or against either internal or external resistance. (Imagine walking through quicksand— this type of resistance definitely feels like extra stuff.) Whenever there is extra anything, the resulting movement is slower, the input higher.

On the other hand, when you move quickly, performing a skill or movement that is familiar without any resistance or load, the input is low. You don't have to think, you can just do it in a fairly automatic (and fast) way.

Imagine you are lifting a barbell. Your brain has to figure out the size of the barbell, how heavy it is, and the best strategy for lifting it up. That's a lot of things, and the extra load is going to impact the timing, sequencing, and coordination of getting it off the floor.

Now imagine after lifting the barbell a few times you do the exact same motion without the barbell. How does it feel?

Light. Fast. Perhaps even effortless.

Without the barbell your brain has no extraneous object or extra weight to navigate. It simply has to figure out the easiest way to make the desired lifting motion.You can move faster without the barbell than you can with the barbell. "The heavy resistance is high input which equals slower output," Adarian said.

So if your goal is to create and train speed, would you use high input or low input?

Low input will teach you how to move fast. High input will teach you how to move slow. Both have a time and place. The one you use depends on the desired output.

Parallel and perpendicular, a complementary pair:

Consider how you use levers to move quickly when you want to go fast, and slowly when you want to linger in the moment. In order to do this, the levers need to have an element of parallel and perpendicular. This creates rotational movement. To briefly recap:

- Perpendicular creates either compression or expansion. Compression creates expansion. Expansion creates compression. Both are input.

- Parallel starts the movement, rotating the lever arm in the direction you want to move. The parallel can be a push-away, a pull towards, a push forward, or a pull in. Without the parallel, there is no way to move. Every movement is rotational movement.

Parallel and perpendicular are how levers work, and since you are a collection of levers, learning how to use parallel and perpendicular to your advantage will alter your movement output.

Establishing and recognizing complementary and adversarial pairs can sometimes feel elusive. It's a search for two things that somehow fit perfectly together and become better together than they are apart. Let's spend a little time looking at complementary pairs that we haven't talked about yet. These complementary pairs can make a big impact on how you move.

Shin-angle change and the thigh, a complementary pair:

Creating movement forward, for most of us, requires movement in the legs. This works because of a dynamic relationship between the shin-angle change and the thigh.

If you want to move fast, the shin has to get out of the way. Learning how to control the shin is a lot like deciding how quickly you want to open a door—the faster you open a door, the faster you can walk through the door. The faster you get the shin out of the way, the faster you move forward.

Whenever you dynamically move your legs, whether it's to walk forward, lunge awkwardly to grab your dog's leash, or carefully pivot your body so you can navigate going down steep terrain, the levers in your legs shift as your anchor points shift. How the levers shift is based on the interplay between the shin angle and the thigh.

Shin angle can be thought of as the rotation between the foot and the shin. The thigh and pelvis are a point of rotation. And what is the joint between the thigh and the shin?

The knee. So another way to think of this is the knee coordinates the movement between the thigh and shin. Think about the person whose torso leans forward in a squat. Are they performing the act of squatting by coordinating the movement from their knee or from their hip?

From their hip. The knee moves second. So the timing, sequencing, and coordination of the movement is going to be impacted. What happens if the same person changes the sequencing and timing so that the knee bends first? Does that change what the squat will look like?

Yes. When you change the timing and the sequencing, you are changing when you are moving the joints with relation to each other and what joints are moving in relation to each other. This means you change the coordination, or how the joints move in relation to each other. And when you change the how, you are changing both the levers that are being used to achieve a specific physical skill and the output, which is the expression of the physical skill.

When you run, your hip joint allows your thigh to rotate forward. This is what swings your leg forward so you can move forward in space. But how does this happen?

It's based on how your foot hits the ground, which is determined by when and what—when the foot hits the ground and what part of the foot hits the ground.

This sets up how the body moves over the foot, which creates the opportunity for the thigh to be extended so that it has space to move into—you need to make space to move into space. As soon as you make space, you are no longer creating compression. Instead, you are generating tension which if you remember from earlier, leads to expansion. This also means the joint has adequate space to allow movement to occur. And how you make space depends on what and when. These three factors, what, when, and how, create the timing, sequencing, and coordination of any movement.

In order for the shin to rotate forward, which two joints create the space for the shin to move into? The ankle and the knee. The shin rotates over the foot and the ankle flexes, allowing the shin to generate a perpendicular force. The knee also flexes, allowing the thigh to rotate. There is a perpendicular relationship between the shin and the thigh that doesn't mean they remain at a ninety-degree angle with each other. Instead, it means the rotation of the thigh maintains a perpendicular action with the shin. This allows the rotational movement of the leg that sends you tumbling forward.

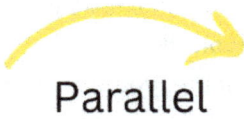

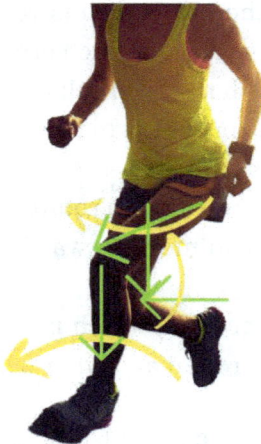

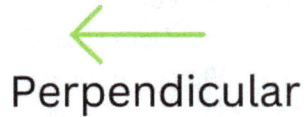

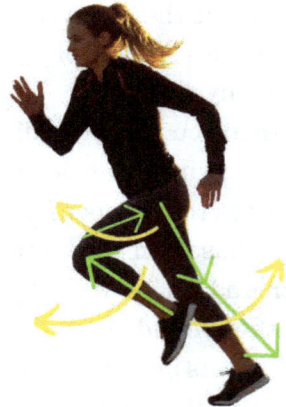

Parallel   Perpendicular

The back and forth between the shin angle and the thigh is a neat reciprocal partnership that dictates how and when the leg moves, how the foot responds to the ground, and how the body is propelled forward.

We keep talking about the rotation that is occurring for the shin to rotate forward, but we're going to switch to the terminology of pitch, yaw, and roll; the threesome you were first introduced to in chapter 3.

It's also one of the threesomes that will be covered later in this chapter. The introduction of these concepts is just that–an introduction to an opportunity for you to begin thinking about movement in a different way.

When your foot is on the ground, your shin pitches, creating rotation in a forward direction.

The foot rolls, rotating to create space for the heel to come up and the body to move forward.

The calf pitches and yaws one way while the thigh pitches and yaws the opposite way. This creates the illusion of the leg staying straight. The rotational movement is what carries the body over the foot and allows the leg to leave the ground and swing forward.

The directions can shift. What I mean by that is the shin pitches forward, and at some point, it might pitch backwards to create the propulsion of the body forward. Or it might pitch forward the entire time as your body tumbles forward over it. Everyone accomplishes movement a little differently. One way isn't better than the other, but learning how you perform certain actions creates an opportunity to try something different. If different is more effective than what you were doing, adopt it and move on. If different doesn't create any marked improvements, chalk the experience up to a fun exploration and go back to what you were doing.

Levers create this neat system of compression and expansion. They work bidirectionally, which means they can speed things up or slow things down.

Imagine a pole vaulter as the pole plants in the box. The pole is initially bent, creating a short lever arm which means it moves fast. The connection between the pole and the ground creates an anchor, and the speed of the bent pole allows the athlete to move up until when?

Until the pole is perpendicular to the ground. It's now a long lever arm, moving more slowly as the athlete moves over the top of the pole. The athlete is the load. The pole is the lever arm. The fulcrum is the pole in the box. When the pole is perpendicular to the ground, the pole acts like another joint for the athlete, which the athlete can use to generate speed and propel their body up and over the bar.

A parallel is maintained between joints, but not to the ground, creating the space to move into that didn't exist previously. Depending on what you are doing, the foot and thigh might be parallel to each other or the torso and shin might be parallel to each other as the body moves forward in space.

When you aren't moving what position is your body in relative to the ground? Perpendicular, just like the pole vault when it isn't moving.

This relationship between the shin and the thigh is generally harmonious, but when it isn't, the joint that is in the middle of these areas, the knee, becomes a sore subject. Foot is on the ground. Shin moves forward (pitch). Lower leg rotates in (yaw). Knee bends. Thigh rotates out (yaw in opposition).

What happens if the lower leg and the thigh yaw in the same direction while the foot is on the ground?

This is nothing you want to actually spend too much time thinking about unless pain is your thing. The knee is a hinge joint, which means it extends the shin forwards and extends the shin backwards (Gupton et al., 2022).

When the lower leg and thigh yaw the same way with the foot on the ground, the knee is going to twist inwards or outwards. Hinges don't withstand twisting well, so this twisting action isn't something to strive for.

Now if your foot rotates inward, pitching, yawing, and rolling, because you are slicing the foot to kick a soccer ball or to go around an obstacle, the entire leg will rotate in that direction. In this example, the foot is dynamically directing the movement of the leg in a 3D rotational movement, not a 2D movement. The response is cooperative, reducing strain throughout the leg so it can respond to the stress being imposed and move.

The knee joint can be flexed when the thigh is flexed. It can also be extended when the thigh is flexed. In fact, the primary muscles that flex and extend the knee are muscles that run along the length of the thigh.

Think of it this way: the thigh and knee are intimately related, which means the thigh and shin are intimately related. The knee is the hinge between the upper and lower legs that allows the leg to move forward in a cohesive way.

The knee joint primarily functions to increase the lever arm of the quadriceps (the muscle group in the front of the thighs) and ensure stability to the entire leg structure under load (Vaienti et al., 2017). Increasing the lever arm, remember, slows things down; shortening the lever arm speeds things up. Another way to think of the knee joint is it allows the leg to move quickly or slowly.

How fast do you move? The answer is largely based on the timing, sequencing, and coordination between the shin angle and the thigh.

How fast you move in general, actually, is based on those three variables. So timing, sequencing, and coordination can be thought of as the first of our threesomes in the world of moving.

Open- and closed-chain movements, a complementary pair:

Something anchors you to the floor, the chair, to another person. Then something else moves, allowing you to move freely, without constraint.

Open-ended movement or open-chain movement refers to whether a limb is moving freely through space, connected only to you, or whether the limb is fixed and you are moving over it, connected to both an outside object and you. For the purposes of this section, you can also think of open-ended movement and closed-ended movement as referring to what is anchored and what isn't.

The most obvious example of this is the leg—if the foot is on the ground and you are moving over the foot, the movement is a closed-chain movement. If your foot is off the ground and your leg is moving through the air, the movement is an open-chain movement (Jewiss et al., 2017).

If you are upside down, walking on your hands, the hands become the anchoring point to the ground. As the hands walk, they are performing a closed-ended movement. The feet are moving freely in the air. They are the open-ended part of the movement.

All movement is a combination of both—you can't have one without the other. The fluidity through which you move from open- to closed-chain movement is all dependent on how smoothly you shift from one anchor point to another. This relates to how you are controlling collisions.

Imagine the basketball player reaching for the ball. He moves from one foot on the ground, to no feet on the ground. His hands reach up between a sea of hands to connect with the desired object.

Once he has the ball, there is a seamless quality to how he rotates his body as his feet land on the ground. He pivots and leaps up, placing the ball in the basket, as he transfers his hands to the rim, hanging for a moment before he returns to the ground.

Can you identify how the anchors shift? What about when different parts of the body are acting as closed-chain joints? What about an open chain?

Now imagine the salsa dancer moving her hips as her feet dance their way towards her partner. She spins as she gets to him. He supports her as she dips down. She turns towards him, their hands locking and unlocking as their bodies turn and rotate, both of their hips moving as their feet tell a story to the music.

Her hips turn again as she extends a leg, wrapping it around his waist. His torso supports her as her hands shift position on his body and her other leg wraps around his leg. She dips back as he supports her with leg and his hands, giving her the appearance of weightlessness, before effortlessly setting her down. Her legs come back to the ground, her arms shift positions, and they begin dancing again.

Can you identify some of the anchor points now on one (or both) of the dancers? What about which movements are closed versus open chain with the arms? What about for the legs?

Quadratus lumborum and scapula, a complementary pair:

What do a professional baseball player and a high-level shot putter have in common?

Let's assume for simplicity's sake that they are both right handed. When they let go of the ball or the shot put, the right scapula for both of them will be fully extended out, away from the spine. This lengthens the arm, allowing the hand to propel the objects as far and as fast as possible.

But what happens on the left side of the back? Something needs to provide an anchor so the right arm can generate speed. Fortunately, the body has a built in solution for this and the left scapula shifts to the right, anchoring into the torso and towards the pelvis via the quadratus lumborum. If the left side didn't provide an anchor, there would be chaos in the torso; chaos isn't conducive to throwing fast.

What else does the anchoring of the left scapula do? It creates compression on the left side, balancing the expansion that is occurring on the right side. When you change the position of your shoulder blade, you change the amount of compression occurring in the torso.

This change in position affects how you use your arms and how you use your feet. While the relationship between the shoulder blade and the pelvis is based on a number of factors, the quadratus lumborum can be thought of as an anchor between the upper body and the pelvis. Because it's difficult to tell where, exactly, it begins, it's not exactly great at producing movement—you could also say this is a muscle that creates compression or acts as an anchor (Bordoni & Varacallo, 2022). It doesn't act as a lever.

What it does do well is act as a crossroads for the forces that are exerted by neighboring muscles. Think of the pitcher and the shot putter. What do they both do after they release the ball and the shot put? They take a step forward. Why? Because the force generated by throwing at such a high speed propels them forward. It takes a minute to slow everything down. One of the things that helps slow things down is the QL, which literally connects the rib cage to the pelvis; which gliding bone rests on the rib cage? The scapula, or shoulder blade.

It's worth noting the upper body is designed to handle external loads while being mobile. This is different from the lower body, which is built

to handle the continual stress from the ground. The spine is a swivel; it can't create an isometric contraction without an isometric load.

What I mean by this is the spine moves through a combination of pitch, yaw, and roll. This is why you can rotate your body through space as you fall towards the ground, pitching down, but also turning and compressing to lessen the impact. We will discuss this more in chapter 6, but a rigid spine is a spine that breaks; a spine that swivels is one that allows you to move freely.

This doesn't mean you always want maximum movement of the spine. You probably don't want a lot of pitching and rolling, for instance, when you are doing a front lever on a pull-up bar. The anchoring of the hands against a solid object changes how much your spine moves.

This is why one way to identify the feeling of isometric contraction through the spine is by holding on to an external object, like a rod or stick. As the object moves through space, there is a response, a corresponding contraction throughout the torso, which might help you find the complementary pairing of the QL and the scapula.

Try this: Place your thumbs around the back of your waist, just above your pelvis, and let the second, third, and fourth fingers wrap around the front of the waist just above the pelvis. Apply some pressure with your fingers inward as you pull the skin down. Imagine you are anchoring the skin of the waist towards the pelvis.

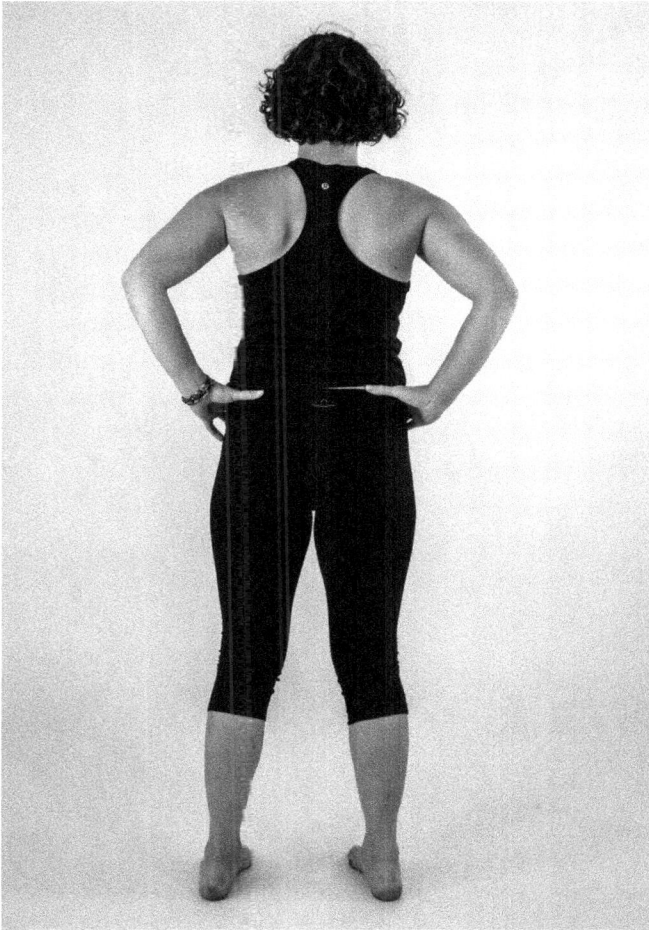

Make some shoulder circles. Feel the movement in the shoulders blades as your shoulders move up and around in a circular direction.

Keep your fingers where they are but stop applying pressure. Make some shoulder circles. Does that feel different? If so, how?

Remove your hands. Create the same action of your fingers, creating an internal pressure down around the sides of your spine. Make shoulder circles. How does that feel?

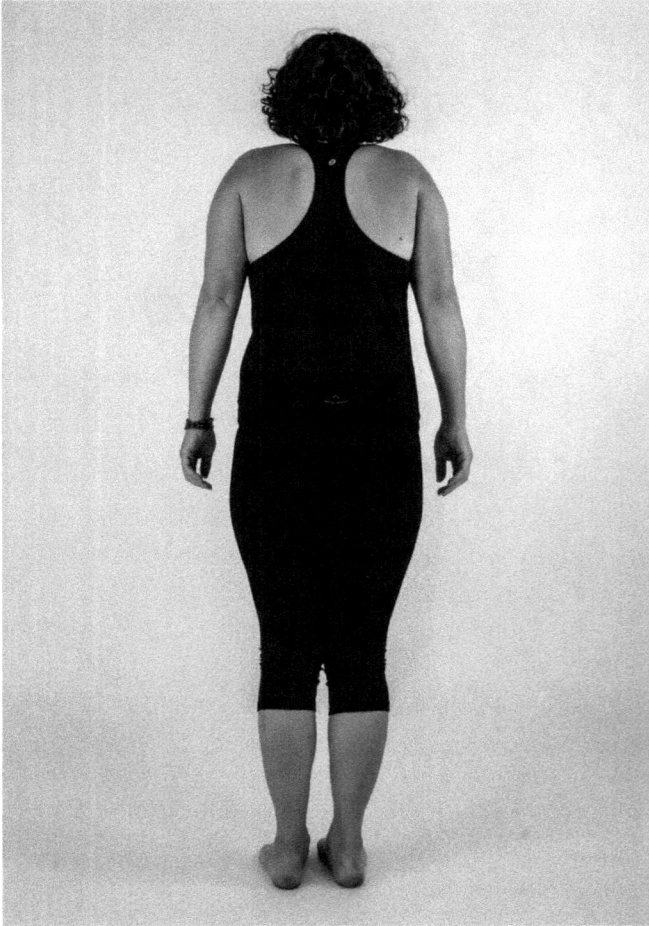

Do the same thing, making shoulder circles without creating internal pressure downward around the sides of your spine. Does that feel different?

When you create a sense of internal pressure, you create a sense of safety because your torso has an anchor. Safety frees up movement. So the QL and the scapula are complementary pairs because the QL allows the scapula to take the brakes off and move without an imminent sense of danger.

Glute and soleus, a complementary pair:

The glute and soleus are complementary pairs. They can work together to rotate the leg.

When the foot is working as a class-two lever, the soleus pulls the heel up and around as the torso rotates over the foot. To complete the rotation of the leg, the gluteal muscles lift and rotate the hip. It creates a cycle of heel lifts foot, then leg swings, lifts, and rotates.

Glute and foot as class-one levers, an adversarial pair:

When the foot acts as a class-one lever as the weight shifts, the glute and soleus no longer complement each other. Instead, there is a conflict. When the torso moves over the foot, instead of the heel lifting up allowing the foot to shift (and becoming a class-two lever and initiating the cycle of the rotation of the leg), the heel stays down. The foot never shifts into a class-two lever, but remains a class-one lever. The heel doesn't lift up until after the weight has passed over the leg.

Why does this matter? Because a class-one lever is more powerful than a class-three lever, but class-three levers are what create speed. In a battle between a class-one lever and a class-three lever, the class-three lever will lose. What does this have to do with class-two levers? The class-two lever creates a strong anchor about the ground so that class-three levers can work. If the foot stays as a class-one lever, it will be good at being strong, but not good at being fast.

It also means the leg can't complete its backward rotation because the glute isn't able to act as a class-three lever to lift the leg backwards. The foot as a class-one lever creates this conflict, preventing rotation. Rotation creates speed. Lack of rotation creates a lack of speed.

The threesomes:

In the movie *Professor Marston and the Wonder Women*, Professor William Marston and his wife, Elizabeth, are a complementary pair, harmoniously working together in the field of psychology. He hires a research assistant, Olive, to aid in the research he was performing in order to develop what would eventually become the lie detector test. William is attracted to Olive, which makes her an adversarial pair for Elizabeth, except Elizabeth is attracted to her, too.

And so a threesome is formed, and that threesome becomes the basis for the character Wonder Woman, which William developed and wrote under a pseudonym until his death at age 62.

This worked because of timing—the Marstons were committed to the development of the lie detector test. Adding Olive was an integral piece in its development.

The timing altered how things were being done both in and out of the laboratory. The sequencing of their professional and personal lives shifted because of the addition of Olive. The university found out about their unique relationship and fired the Marstons (this was the late 1920s/ early 1930s).

The conceptualization of the character Wonder Woman was predicated by this entire sequence of events involving an unusual pair which became a threesome. If you can find the pairs, you can begin to identify how they dance together to create the elements of movement; the movement that occurs because of triads in a complex way.

Pitch, yaw, and roll: A review

Pitch, yaw, and roll are a threesome that we discussed earlier, a triad of actions that describe the six degrees of freedom a rigid body has while moving in a three-dimensional space ("Pitch, yaw," 2022). They were introduced in chapter 2, but let's view them more concretely using the concepts we have explored so far.

In order to pitch, what needs to happen? Remember, pitch is what happens when the head nods up and down, the torso moves forward or backwards, or the foot moves down or up. The center shifts forward or backwards—towards the earth or away from the earth. The ability of different segments of the body (think joints) to pitch, yaw, and roll depends on how the joints are interacting with each other.

Think about the baseball pitcher from earlier. When he winds up to pitch the ball, he yaws his torso towards the ball and rolls his arm back. As he brings the ball up and around, he pitches his body forward, yaws his torso away from the ball, and rolls his hips. The interplay between pitch, yaw, and roll is determined by how and when the joints produce movement—the levers are the output and provide the input, which causes the next output.

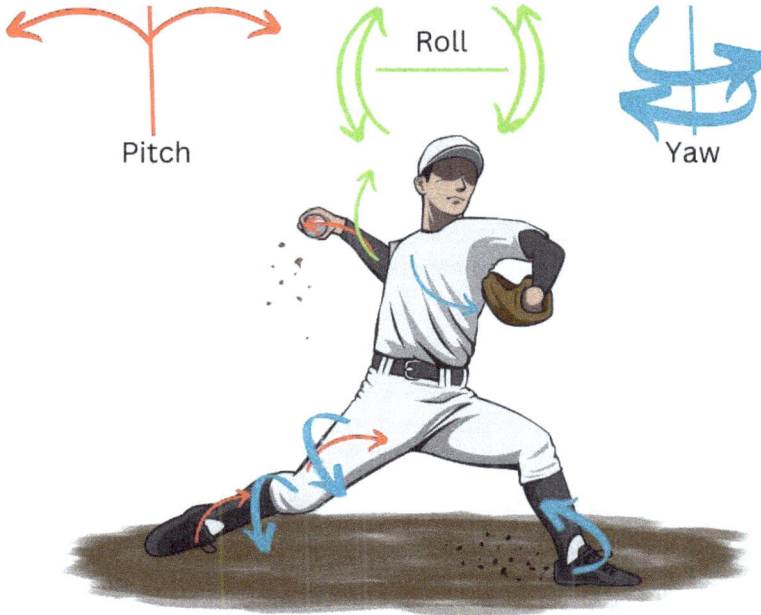

What would happen if the pitcher's body didn't yaw towards the ball as he was winding up the ball? The roll of the arm would be affected. How the roll would be affected depends on a number of factors, like whether he pitches his body back or whether he rolls his hip. Pitch, yaw, and roll are an expression of timing, sequencing, and coordination which are determined by what, how, and when. (Threesomes in this section abound.)

Pitch is a way to balance the body as it moves through space (Ristroph et al., 2013). Think about that for a moment—in order to move, there is a change in orientation of some or all of the body parts. The pitch is what prevents the body from being knocked off-balance every single time you move.

If you toss a heavy object forward with all of your strength, what happens? The momentum from the toss forces you to take a step forward. Your body pitches forward in space, your neuromuscular system anticipates the change in body position and adjusts accordingly.

Or, you could flip everything so that the pitch is reversed. This is what happens in a hip thrust. The weight provides the input that pushes the hips down. The output is the thrust upward, which is a reverse pitch of the body.

Our legs prevent us from tumbling forward or doing a forward roll every time we change our pitch. The pitch of the body is partially what determines how the legs move underneath us. Shin-angle change becomes a function of how far our torso pitches forward. The resulting lever arms determine how quickly the legs move underneath us.

Yaw is the movement of the head when it shakes slowly back and forth, opposing a specific thought or idea. How do you know where your body is positioned in space? The ability to dynamically balance comes, in large part, from the inner ear, which gets information from position-dependent gravity cues (Vimal et al., 2018). Another way to think of this is how you are moving (or the output) influences the input which influences the output. (The circle of moving→sensing→moving→sensing is a constant interplay in everything you do. If you haven't noticed this pattern, which would be hard since I keep bringing it up, take note of it now.)

Anyway, you can pitch and yaw at the same time. If I lean my torso forward as I rotate my right ear to my left knee, I am pitching the torso and yawing the head. Or, if I lean forward at the ankles as I place my right and then left hand next to my right foot so that I can enter into a handstand, I am pitching the entire body forward and yawing the torso to the right.

Which brings me to roll, the action of ambivalently taking the right ear to the right shoulder or the left ear to the left shoulder. Roll tips the body sideways, allowing you to cartwheel or do a jumping jack. Pitch and yaw are complemented by roll to allow the body to turn and rotate, like throwing a ball at a high speed or catching your footing so you don't fall.

Imagine you are out running and you catch your right foot on a rock. Your right leg twists underneath you. Your body rotates and leans to the left as your torso leans forward until your right foot lands on the ground in front of you.

What just happened?

The right leg yaws and rolls under you when you catch your right foot on the rock. Your body rolls and yaws to the left in an effort to counterbalance the right foot. The torso pitches forward, allowing the right foot to swing forward so you stay upright.

What are the anchor points? What are some of the lever arms?

Hopefully, you are starting to see that pitch, yaw, and roll can act alone. You can pitch the body forward, with no yaw or roll anywhere else. This is a unidirectional action, one that involves no rotation in any other joint.

Do you remember the kiss from chapter 2, when I asked if you preferred kissing someone head-on or if you preferred to rotate the head as your lips meet? This example was used to illustrate collisions, but it is also a great example of 1D versus 2D movement. 1D movement involves less coordination. It lacks finesse, which means the resulting stress and strain aren't always complementary.

This may be why people who move in a 1D way get hurt—this unidirectional way of moving results in a lot of strain in one area. When you move in a 2D or 3D way, injuries can still happen, but the collision is managed better. You are less likely to run your nose into your partner's nose when you lean forward to receive a kiss. The rotation of the head allows the stress and strain to be more complementary, resulting in a less stressful experience.

The arms of your partner embrace you as you rotate your body to the right. You attempt to wrap your feet under and to the left of their hips to give yourself some leverage. You flex your hips backward, moving your belly away from theirs as you try and wiggle your way out of their grasp.

Your body yaws to the right. Your legs are yawing and rolling to the left. Your hips pitch backward in an effort to eventually break free.

What are the anchor points? What are some of the lever arms? The movement is a 3D movement involving elements of pitch, yaw, and roll that reduces the stress imposed upon you as you move.

You step your right foot on a stool while holding the world's most obscure pot in your left hand. You push off your left foot as you reach the pot up and to the right, trying to place it back into its appropriate corner on the top shelf.

Your body pitches forward when you step the right foot on the stool. As you push off the left foot, your body pitches forward, and yaws and rolls to the right. Your left arm pitches forward and yaws to the right.

What are the anchor points? What are some of the lever arms?

Stress, strain, and deformation: A preview

There is one more threesome that we have touched upon throughout these pages. Stress, strain, and deformation are the threesome that explains the relationship between something, the response to that something, and the result of that response..

Stress is the something. Stress can be external (gravity, a heavy box of books, a barbell). It can be internal (fatigue, illness, soreness). Stress knocks things away from homeostasis.

Whenever there is stress, there is an internal response. This internal response is strain.

When you are sick, what happens? You are achy and sore. Your entire system feels off. The virus that has invaded your body creates a strain that you can feel.

What is the response to that strain? Your immune system kicks into high gear, mobilizing all kinds of cells to combat the invader. These cells aren't usually needed, so their presence creates a deformation internally. This deformation is movement.

When you walk downhill, gravity creates stress, pulling your foot towards the ground. To prevent your foot from crashing into the hillside, there is strain to slow the foot down. The foot landing against the ground is the deformation. It is the result of the stress and strain working together, which creates a movement.

When you pick up a heavy box of books, the weight of the box creates stress on your arms and your torso. Your body responds with strain in your muscles and ligaments so you don't drop the box of books. How you shift while you are holding (and supporting) the box of books is the deformation.

We will cover stress, strain, and deformation more fully in chapter 6, but for now, just know they are an important threesome in the world of movement.

Complementary pairs, adversarial pairs, and threesomes begin to fill-in the lines of how moving occurs during different activities and everyday life. As we move into our final chapter on flexibility and mobility, think about the different complementary pairs and threesomes. Where do they fit? How is the body navigating space through pitch, yaw, and roll? What is the what, how, and when of the move? Can you identify the stress and the strain? What is the resulting deformation?

CHAPTER 6

DROP IT LIKE IT'S LITERAL, DEFINING TERMS

A leg encircles yours. You rotate, feeling the weight of the leg shift up, towards your hip. As the pressure shifts on your hip, you lean into the pressure a little more, establishing a longer collision, the vibration from the leg gently pulsing through you.

We have talked about a number of ways to help you on your way to experiencing elation during movement. Elation is accompanied by the freedom to flow, allowing you to lengthen and rotate, spin and compress and expand. The result is the ability to navigate pressure and the accompanying vibrations and collisions that occur every time you move.

This final chapter before all of the exercises explores common words that are used when describing humans as they move. Can you improve your flexibility to be more bendy? Should you improve your stiffness to generate more force? Can you move your joints in a variety of ways? Is your structure stable?

These are the questions that are commonly asked, but step back for a moment and ask yourself how useful are these questions, really? Do the words used accurately describe a person moving through space in a way that is fast and coordinated, or slow and graceful? (Or fast and graceful and slow and coordinated?) Is the sequencing, coordination, and timing required to execute a specific motor task actually described with words like flexibility, stiffness, stability, or articulation?

We have frequently referenced the idea that compression + expansion + vibration + pressure = elation. Compression, expansion, vibration, and pressure are all things that stress the system. Elation is the strain on the system.

We discussed the threesome of stress, strain, and deformation earlier, but they are important enough to be explored more deeply.

Stress is any and all force imposed upon you. Many things can be considered stress. When you barbell squat, for instance, what are some of the sources of stress?

There's gravity, pulling you down towards the ground. The barbell adds an external force, and depending on its position, how you navigate the stress through the levers of your limbs will vary. There's internal compression, which corresponds with an increase in blood pressure.

Stress is an input, so any stress imposed will affect output.

Stress can be low, like when you stand with both feet against the ground. It can be high, like when you pull your pinky finger backward towards your wrist or when you perform a heavy barbell squat.

Stress creates strain. Movement is the deformation.

Strain is the resistance to the imposed stress or force. To strain is to resist force. When you stand with both feet on the ground, you produce enough internal strain so you don't fall over.

In the barbell squat example above, what are some of the ways you strain?

Your leg muscles strain, resisting the pull of gravity. The muscles in your torso strain, resisting the compression from the weight. Your arteries strain, resisting the increase in pressure on the circulatory system.

Like stress, strain can be low or it can be high. When you are standing with two feet on the ground, the amount of stress is low and the resulting strain is low. When you pull your pinky finger backward towards your wrist, the stress is high and the strain on the knuckle is high, preventing the finger from pulling so far back that it breaks.

And when you barbell squat, the stress and strain are both high as the force on the system competes with the resistance to the force.

Imagine the yogi, who is bending into a deep backbend. There is stress occurring from gravity and enough strain to not flop into the position, but not so much strain that the back doesn't deeply bend.

Imagine trying to touch your toes with straight legs. The stress comes from gravity as you fold your body into a position that may or may not be comfortable. If there is a lot of strain, how close do you think you get to your toes?

Not very. The strain causes you to resist the movement down towards your feet, making your toes feel very far away.

Stress and strain are complementary pairs, with one influencing the other to create the optimal amount of movement and tension.

The amount of deformation that occurs depends on the tug of war between stress and strain. When the strain is enough to counteract the stresses being imposed, the shape doesn't change very much (if at all). This momentary standoff between stress and tension results in an isometric contraction—even though there is tension, there is no movement.

When you think about a movement you want to perform, ask yourself this: Where do I want the movement to occur? How can I control it?

The adventures of Gumby and Mr. Robot:

The character Gumby folds easily, bending into a variety of positions without resisting the stress imposed upon him. If he is pulled or folded too much, he isn't able to return to his original shape. It doesn't take much for Gumby to become plastic and permanently deformed, his shape forever altered. Gumby isn't very elastic and struggles to balance stress with strain.

Mr. Robot, on the other hand, doesn't move easily. It moves in a 1D way with a set amount of tension, unable to generate more or less. With the right amount of stress, it moves forward in a way that looks different from how you or I move. When the stress gets to be too much for the robot, it tips over, unable to return to its original position. The robot is more elastic than Gumby, but less elastic than you.

One final note on stress, strain, and deformation before we move into flexibility—stress and strain, like deformation, aren't one-dimensional. They work in a multidimensional way, which is why the resulting movement is usually a combination of pitch, yaw, and roll. Stress—and the resulting strain—can happen from many different angles. If you want to learn to create strain in a variety of ways, isometric contractions give you an opportunity to feel stress, create strain in a multidimensional way, and observe where strain needs to be released in order to facilitate a specific deformation. What strain needs to be released to allow the shin to rotate forward? What strain prevents rotation in the scapula? What happens when you release that strain?

After slowing things down to feel the prevention and facilitation of deformation, go move fast. Implement the concepts in a dynamic way. See what happens.

As you think about concepts like flexibility and stiffness, ask yourself: What is the stress? What is the strain? If I change the stress or the strain, do I get closer to the response I am seeking?

Flexibility: An aspiration for many

Flexibility is a noun, a word that is synonymous with resiliency, elasticity, and being limber. Something that is flexible is pliant, or yielding (Merriam-Webster, n.d.) According to Dictionary.com (n.d.), flexibility is an attribute that implies an object "bends easily or without breaking."

Flexibility is synonymous with resiliency. A flexible system is an adaptable system, one that can fluidly adjust when the current strategy isn't working. Flexibility, then, leads to a sense of strength.

Though the word limber is considered synonymous with the word flexible, it actually has a slightly different definition, one that might more accurately describe what is commonly being sought when people begin flexibility training. Limber is an adjective that specifically refers to a person's mind or body part and means lithe or supple. Merriam-Webster (n.d.) defines limber as "having a supple and resilient quality (as of mind or body): agile, nimble."

In fitness and athletics, flexibility generally refers to muscle stiffness or tension. In order to quantify flexibility, it has become a word that is often used to reference the amount of usable range of motion at a joint. It is also generally believed that in order to increase the range of motion available, a fitness intervention such as stretching should be used to increase the length of intrinsic properties, like the connection point between the muscles and tendons (Pate et al., 2012).

But when you contrast the word flexibility with the word limber, which more accurately describes a desired quality for movement?

Here is the thing about flexibility, which we are using to describe the experience of whether you move freely or stiffly in an area: it has less to do with the length of any of your muscles or tendons and more to do with sensory input. Actually, scratch that—because you don't really want to change the length of your muscles and tendons (they are designed to fit neatly between two bones for a reason). Flexibility doesn't have anything to do with muscle and tendon length, but everything to do with input.

Consider the following scenario: You are walking into a movie theater. It's dark. The trailers have already started and you are waiting for your eyes to adjust so you can find a seat.

You begin walking, slowly, aware that the aisle is sloping downwards.

Suddenly, you feel a hand gripping your right arm. You startle, catching your left toe against the floor.

You fall down, the grip on your arm releasing. Do you think your body is stiff or relaxed as you hit the ground?

Now imagine this: You are sitting in a hot tub on a deck, after a massage. It's nighttime, the stars shine brightly, and the moon is half-full. In the distance, you can see the faintest trace of mountains.

You stand up, and begin navigating your body out of the hot tub. As your right foot hits the ground on the deck, you feel a little light-headed.

You step your left foot forward to catch you, but it doesn't support your weight. You gently collapse, landing on the ground.

Are you more or less stiff when you hit the ground in this scenario? If someone were to measure your hamstring flexibility directly after both of these situations, in which situation would they be more flexible?

In most people, they would be more flexible after the massage and hot tub debacle. Why? Because even though in this hypothetical situation you fell, you were in a safe environment. The sensory input from the previous activities (touch from the massage, the warm water from the hot tub, and the visually pleasing natural setting) doesn't tell your body that it needs to be on guard against anything. And so, you (and your muscles) will be more relaxed.

Because that's the thing about flexibility—the sensory input the brain receives from the environment and the body determines how safe it is for joints to move into certain positions (Guissard & Duchateau, 2006; Behm et al., 2013). In the movie theater example, nothing about the situation was safe; from the dark, unknown environment, to the unsolicited grasp of the arm. The body responds accordingly, tensing against the unknown.

This can be observed in a variety of ways. After a massage, people often report feeling looser or less stiff; these feelings have been measured as actual increases in flexibility (Kaur & Sinha, 2020).

Stretching regularly corresponds to flexibility improvements (at least initially). While there may be an observable change in how flexible you are, those changes are largely due to things like getting used to the sensation of the stretch or getting more comfortable being in the position that initially felt tight.

If you are like me, the first time you drive somewhere new, you plug it into your phone, and then let the phone tell you when to turn left and how many miles it is until your exit. You have no internal map of the location, so you have to rely on an external one. This maybe creates a little bit of anxiety because you aren't sure how to get where you are going, and have no sense of how it relates to other places you have been.

As you get closer to your final destination, you have to be careful not to miss the address. Even though the phone tells you the destination is on your left, unless you are moving slowly, reading addresses, or looking for a sign, it's easy to drive right past your stopping point.

Slowing down and carefully looking is what your brain does when your body approaches a position it doesn't recognize. There is an assessment period as the brain determines whether the feedback it is getting from the joint (or joints) means the position is safe. Anything that is new always takes a moment, a pause while the brain takes all of the new sensory input and accumulates it together to determine the appropriate output. (Or, in the case of our phone mapping example, the pause is the slowing down to look for the address.)

The next time you drive to the same location, you might still need to rely on your phone to get there, but you won't have to slow down as much to find the turn. And each subsequent trip will result in more familiarity, with less and less reliance on the phone to navigate until, eventually, the route is comfortable.

The same thing happens with repeated exposure to a position that is initially new—as familiarity increases, so does comfort level, until the position no longer causes enough sensory input to send off potential warning signs. The corresponding output is a position that has more range.

But (there's always a but), this interesting thing happens when you watch high-level athletes who aren't focused on controlling or achieving a specific range of motion—the nature of their sport creates the environment for them to achieve large amounts of flexibility.

Someone recently posted a video of the fastest-baseball infield throw of the season (it's 2022 as of this writing). It was thrown by the shortstop to the first baseman and clocked at ninety-seven miles per hour. What, perhaps, was more impressive than the speed of the throw, was the catch made by the athlete playing first base. His legs were in an extremely wide straddle, almost a side splits. He caught the ball in that position, popped right out of it, and threw the ball back to the pitcher. Impressive.

The stress comes from gravity. The strain is the body resisting gravity. The deformation is the legs moving into a splits position.

When the first baseman initially moved into the splits position to catch the ball, there was a lot of stress and a lot of strain. This allowed maximal deformation (movement) without his legs popping out of his hip socket. Once he was in the splits position, there was a lot of stress and a lot of strain to prevent any further deformation—he was at the end point of his range.

What would have happened if his hip had popped out of its socket?

He wouldn't have been able to stand back up. At least not easily. There would have been a change in the tendons and ligaments around the hip. Instead of being in a state of elasticity, the structures that hold the hip in place would have become permanently deformed.

A material whose shape is altered in a lasting way is in a state of plasticity, which is the opposite of elasticity. This means if the structures in his hip permanently deformed, they can no longer return to their original shape unless they are repaired through medical intervention. They are permanently changed.

If you break one of the bones in your arm, your arm is placed in a cast. The broken bone is in a state of plasticity; it is placed in a cast so it has an opportunity to heal and return to a state of elasticity.

Play-Doh is elastic when you initially pull it apart. If you were to stop pulling on it, it would return to its original shape.

At some point, if you pull hard enough, it breaks. The broken piece is changed in a perpetual way. It's less strong, the structure not able to withstand high amounts of stress.

If you want the broken piece of Play-Doh to become strong again, you reintegrate it with the rest of the Play-Doh so it can once again be in an elastic state.

When pulled taut, a strand of curly hair will return to its curly shape when it's no longer being pulled. It's elastic. If you straighten the strand of curly hair with a flat iron, it becomes plastic. If you pull the now straightened hair follicle more taut, it breaks. The act of straightening the curl causes a change in the mechanical makeup of the hair follicle. Something that is plastic is something that has changed shape in a permanent way.

Let's return to our first baseman. Does the first baseman need to stretch in order to achieve maximal elasticity? Or does he just need to play (and practice) a lot of baseball?

The truth about stiffness and muscles:

Stiff is a weird word. Synonyms for stiff include arthritic, creaky, and rigid (Thesaurus.com, n.d.). Muscular stiffness, which is synonymous with muscular elasticity or resistance to stretch, is actually desirable (Nichols & Huyghues-Despointes, 2009). A muscle that has a high degree of elasticity is one that resists stretch (Roberts, 2016).

But (and there's always a but) the truth about muscular stiffness is it's contradictory to the dictionary definition of muscular stiffness. This leaves the entire conversation around the topic of stiffness in a vague and confusing place. Is it good? Is it bad? How much is too much? How little is too little? If I am rigid and arthritic I feel stiff, but now you are saying if I don't easily stretch I am stiff and that is actually a good thing?

It's enough to make you feel dizzy while you try and make sense of it all.

Rather than be vague and confusing (which sends mixed messages), we are striving for clear and concise. In order to be clear and concise we are going to describe a muscle that is elastic as a muscle with residual muscle tension.

In the effort of full disclosure, this isn't a phrase we just made up. It is actually a technical term that is used to define the tone of the muscle at rest (Madhok & Shabbir, 2022).

Think about this—if you are relaxed and lounging on the couch, are your muscles fully relaxed and contracted at all?

No. If this were the case, your skeleton would have no form. You would be an unformed shape. Your muscles have a residual tone or tension that keeps your shape.

What happens if you are lounging on the couch and you have a lot of tension in your low back? This high amount of tension makes it difficult to get comfortable. Is the residual muscle tension higher or lower than it needs to be for you to perform the act of lounging on the couch?

It's higher than it needs to be, which means there is a lot of strain for a low stress situation.

What if you are laying on the couch and you are having a difficult time getting comfortable because your body doesn't feel supported? You feel floppy, like you need more support. What does this suggest about your residual muscle tension?

In this situation, the residual muscle tension is lower than is optimal for the stress of couch lounging. This isn't an uncommon situation for people with a lot of stretch in their ligaments, the fibrous structures that connect bone to bone. Ligaments aren't supposed to stretch very much because you don't want a lot of space between bones. Too much space means not very much pressure.

Remember how pressure provides input and input determines output? Compression creates pressure. Ligaments have very little stretch, which means they get lots of information about the pressure and compression in the joints. A loose ligament means there is less pressure in the joint. This results in less input.

The result?

Less residual muscle tension to hold the structure up. Sometimes the result is too much residual muscle tension in certain parts of the body to make up for too little residual muscle tension in other parts of the body.

Too little residual muscle tension means there isn't enough strain to match the stress.

But what about the movement?

Imagine a thick elastic band. Does it stretch more or less easily than a thin elastic band?

Less easily. Which means it takes more stress to strain the thick rubber band versus the thin rubber band.

What does this have to do with movement? When you actually stress the thick rubber band, the rubber strains and the shape deforms. When you remove the stress, what happens?

The rubber band quickly returns to its original shape. So having a higher degree of elasticity will result in a faster movement when stress is removed.

Stress, strain, and bones: When the stress is too much to bear

Bones are a good example of a physiological structure that are designed to withstand high amounts of stress. When compression from external stress is higher than the bone's internal strain, the bone can't maintain its elasticity. It breaks, fracturing. If you fall on an outstretched arm and land with all of your weight on your wrist, your wrist compresses. If the load is too much for your wrist, the radius, one of the bones in your forearm, breaks from the compressive stress.

When a bone isn't regularly stressed in a way that is tolerated, it becomes weaker and less able to create internal strain. This makes it more susceptible to breaking from compression. This happens when astronauts go to space, people are on prolonged bed rest, or when someone doesn't regularly move their body in a variety of ways.

Bones also break when they are moved in opposite directions. If you place your hands together like they are clapping and then move your right hand up as you move the left one down, they slide past each other. If you experience some sort of unexpected high impact, like a car accident or crashing after you jump out of an airplane and your parachute doesn't deploy, the stress from impact will likely be more than certain parts of the skeleton can withstand. The internal strain won't be enough to prevent the sliding, or shearing action, of the bone. There will be a deformation that isn't exactly permanent because bone is a living tissue. It will heal with time, though not in the exact same way as before.

What about muscle cramps?

A muscle cramp, which is sometimes attributed to high muscle tone, actually originates from the nerves that innervate muscles (Miller & Layer, 2005). The exact reason you get an intense muscle cramp isn't exactly clear, though it can be related to lots of things, like the nerve cells being overly excited, and the physiology of the cell membrane (Swash et al., 2019). One way to alleviate the sensation associated with a muscle cramp is to stretch the cramping muscle. This probably makes the nerve cells less excited because of the effect stretching has on a specific type of nerve cell embedded in the junction between muscles and tendons called the Golgi tendon organ (Bordoni et al., 2022; Giuriato et al., 2018).

If the goal isn't to reduce muscle tone and you aren't experiencing that unparalleled sensation caused by muscle cramping, why stretch at all? And what is the goal if you are focused primarily on movement freedom?

"We want to train on the edge of our elasticity," says Adarian.

You lift your leg a little higher, letting your back reach up and arch slightly, your hands gently braced against the floor. You pause for a moment, embracing the sensation, before shifting to find a different position.

Babies do this all of the time, as they use the floor to provide input for the skin, muscles, and joints. As the baby makes their way through the birth canal, they must scrunch, rotate, and extend in order to make their entrance into the world (Medline Plus, 2022). Once they have arrived, they immediately begin working on building the strength to move away from the ground, trying a variety of positions until they successfully figure out how to do things like roll over, sit up, stand, and walk. This strength building doesn't just impact the muscles; the shape of a baby's spine changes significantly until age five, from a C-shape to the S-shape that is associated with the curve in the small of the back. This curve is also known as the lordotic curve and is developed through things like standing, walking, and running (Saunders et al., 2020).

The baby's quest for strength requires getting longer in order to move up. Babies are constantly testing their range, exploring how far they can reach and how that reaching impacts their ability to move. Maybe the goal of the adult human isn't necessarily to stretch and achieve large degrees of range at each joint; rather, the goal is, perhaps, to be able to lengthen and fold. Can you get long? Can you fold up small? Can you do this with each limb? What is your range?

Before we move on, we should note that yes, if you are training or doing things like wrapping a leg around a pole while the other leg is nestled up on your shoulder, or moving from your stomach to your hands with your feet off the ground and back to your stomach regularly, you are going to need more range than someone whose main activities involve cooking dinner and walking to the mailbox. If you are a person that is regularly moving your body into positions that are more expansive than most of the population, you could benefit from training that emphasizes your range.

Remember from earlier that usually when people talk about stiffness they are referring to joint stiffness, not muscle stiffness. The experience of feeling stiff is generally related to an inability to move freely. Movement, remember, occurs because of rotation at a joint, and joints are a hotbed of sensory information. When the brain gets information from the cells in the joint that less rotation can happen or that there is something restricting about the way the bones are currently positioned it is translated into a feeling of stiffness. Joints provide sensory input as part of proprioception. Based on that input, the output is determined.

If we return to the idea that stress creates strain and movement is the response, then it should make sense that one way to change the sensory input is to change the focal point of the movement.

Imagine you were going to punch a punching board. What is the most effective way to do this?

Now imagine you were going to punch something less stiff, like a friend you like to spar with. Would your punch look different?

Yes, for a few different reasons, one of which is that these two situations require different amounts of tension in the arm. When you punch a board, finishing with a bent elbow prevents recoil in the upper body. Recoil is akin to vibration. Too much recoil will knock you down. To minimize unwanted vibrations, you finish the punch with a bent elbow.

Contrast this to sparring with your friend. In order to create the biggest impact, you land your punch with a locked elbow, creating as much tension as possible. Your friend is (hopefully) trying to get out of the way of the punch, so you accelerate forward into the punch (which is what happens when you finish with a straight elbow) while your friend attempts to slow down the acceleration and get out of the way. The pressure that results from the contact of your hand with your friend is the stress; how your friend responds will determine the amount of strain on your system.

When the arm isn't locked out it moves faster. Why? Because shorter levers are for speed. The shorter the arm, the faster it will go.

If we stay with the punching example, different punches are used for different things, largely because of how fast the arm moves. When you throw an uppercut, your arm moves fast. The elbow stays bent the entire time, so the arm is short. This allows you to be quick with both the punch and your response to the punch. The arm will be tense the entire time, minimizing strain and deformation.

The minimal strain that occurs as the arm moves rapidly through the air happens because of the stress from gravity, internal pressure, and compression.

If you throw an overhand punch, the arm is much longer, the elbow not as bent. This means the arm will move slower.

When you land the punch, there will be deformation, making the punch more impactful.

In both scenarios, gravity creates stress. The strain is the resistance to gravity and to the impact from the target. The amount of strain determines the amount of deformation.

In the uppercut, the arm strains to keep the elbow bent as it moves through the air and connects with a hard board. The hard board isn't pliable, so it resists the blow from your hand, causing less deformation or movement. If the board were soft rather than hard, when your hand connected there would be a lot of deformation (movement).

High elasticity leads to low deformation. Low elasticity leads to high deformation.

What happens if there is too much deformation?

There is a tipping point. The tipping point is when you move into a state of plasticity.

When you land each punch, there is stress as your hand collides with its target. The reverberation from the collision creates strain. The stress creates vibrations and pressure. The result of the stress and strain is the deformation.

Adarian explained it like this, "Stress is any and all forces. Strain is the resistance to the anything."

Imagine you are doing a Jefferson curl. There is lots of stress (gravity, external load), but it's low strain because you aren't resisting the pull downwards.

The result?

Lots of deformity as your torso folds over your legs.

Contrast this with a backbend. There is a lot of stress as you bend backwards.

There is a lot of resistance as your torso resists bending backwards.

The result?

A lot of stress, a lot of strain, but (for most of us) little deformity because the spine can only bend so far back.

Different combinations of stress and strain result in different amounts of deformation. Remember, the deformation is the movement and is dependent on whether an area has high or low elasticity.

What does all of this mean with regards to flexibility training? Maybe we should think about flexibility training differently. Maybe flexibility training is actually range training.

A quick detour to the Achilles tendon:

The Achilles tendon is the strongest tendon in the human body. It connects the plantaris, gastrocnemius, and soleus to the heel bone (Pabón & Naqvi, 2022).

For the Achilles to be strong, it must also be elastic, which, remember from above, means it resists deformity.

Now imagine you are hell-bent on keeping your heels down in a squat because you were told that's how you are supposed to squat. What happens to the Achilles?

It deforms, but the Achilles is passive.

Contrast this with allowing the heels to come up when you squat. What happens?

The Achilles still deforms, but it becomes more tense, functioning more like a rod.

The same is true in a split-stance position. If you don't actively press the ball of the back of the foot into the ground as the heel comes up, the back Achilles deforms passively. If you force the front of the heel to stay on the ground in a split stance position, the front Achilles deforms passively.

What does this mean for movement? If the goal is maximal, passive deformation of the Achilles, then keep your heels down when you squat. If the goal is to train to move fast or dynamically, let your heels lift.

This isn't unlike the arches of the feet. When the arches are formed, the foot becomes more taut, allowing the foot to propel you forward quickly. When the foot leaves the ground, the arches are no longer needed, and the foot becomes passive.

The Achilles acting as a rod contributes to how you use your foot because the tension pulls on things, creating a secondary deformity. One thing leads to another. Just like the Achilles passively deforming contributes to how you use your foot.

Back to flexibility and range:

Range means lots of things, but in this context, the range is the distance or extent between possible extremes.

The overhand punch required more range than the uppercut punch. Why?

Because in this example, range refers to the distance the arm moves between the starting position and the end position. The overhand punch required maximal distance; the uppercut is dependent on minimal distance and maximal speed.

Stiffness, remember, is related to a stiff joint, and as a result the range is determined by the sensory input from the joints and the tension in the muscles.

When you sprain an ankle or have changes inside the joint, like osteoarthritis or a cyst, the nervous system will receive sensory input that creates stiffness.

This stiffness creates resistance to movement, minimizing deformation.

If you don't have an acute injury or osseous changes such as osteoarthritis or a cyst, what should you think about when you consider range training?

Ask yourself if there is resistance where you want resistance when you move.

Work on controlling the range you have. Train at the edge of your elasticity.

If you consistently train past the edge of your elasticity, you might impact your tipping point, lowering it. And if you lower your tipping point, you become less resilient and more likely to move from elastic to plastic.

If you need more range for a specific activity (like pole dancing), work on your range by figuring out where there is resistance or strain, and where there isn't. How can you adjust the stress and the strain to create the movement you want?

Keep in mind that when you approach end range of a position, you have the ability to create less tension than when you are in mid-range. The baseball player whose legs were at end range when he caught the ball is going to create less tension in his legs when he moves from that position than the boxer whose legs are underneath them, knees bent, feet moving quickly. Short levers, remember, are stronger than long levers.

What also happens when a joint is at end range? The joint becomes "locked" to prevent twisting. Think of this as the joint becoming secure and having less available movement.

If you focus on range training instead of flexibility training, what does it look like? Does it look like traditional flexibility training? Does twisting your body up like a pretzel work on the range you need to do the things you want to do?

Maybe your range training actually looks a lot like practicing the positions you are going to be regularly using in a thoughtful way.

Imagine this: You are an inflexible twenty-something who can't even touch your toes. So you start doing yoga, because yoga is supposed to make you more flexible.

You do yoga three times a week, because even though you aren't getting more flexible, you are pretty sure this yoga thing is supposed to be magical in some way and one day, you are certain, you are going to be able to easily touch the floor.

After ten years, you realize you still aren't as flexible as you want to be (yes, it takes ten years in this imaginary scenario for you to figure out the input isn't creating the desired output). You stop yoga and start tumbling and doing different types of acrobatics based activities. And guess what? Your range improves dramatically and you are actually able to do the things you had always wanted to do.

Why did this work with minimal static stretching?

Because the input is the output. The input is always enough to influence the output, so if the input never changes, the output is never going to change. To put this another way: if the intervention isn't teaching the entire system to develop strength and safety in that specific position in order to better tolerate the resulting collisions, there will be no adaptation to the intervention. Or maybe there will be, but you might not like it. Your brain prioritizes safety—if it doesn't like what you are doing, the output might not be what you desire.

A quick side note—range is about collision, flexion, or extension. The amount of range you use is predicated by these three things.

When Galen Rupp, one of the fastest male long-distance runners in the US as of this writing, is running at a high speed, the muscles in his leg continue moving his leg back as his foot is preparing to leave the ground, while his torso moves forward. The muscles create the end range position.

When his foot hits the ground, there is a collision. The ankle responds, flexing, moving into its end range. The collision creates the range.

As he moves over the front leg and the leg flexes, the muscles in his leg moves his torso over his leg. The muscles create the range.

Another way to think of it is like this: his foot collides with the ground, causing joints to flex. His leg tensions, so he doesn't end up collapsed on the ground from the impact. He moves over his leg, the leg becomes less tense, and the muscles create more range as his foot leaves the ground.

If you keep these three concepts in mind (collision, flexion, and extension) and you remember that muscles or a collision create flexion or extension, options for maximizing your range may begin to unveil themselves to you. (And if not, don't worry. There are lots of ideas in the next section.)

You can also think about Rupp's running gait from the perspective of stress, strain, and deformation. When his foot collides with the ground, there is stress and strain occurring from two places: gravity and the ground. His ankle responds to this bidirectional stress and strain dynamically flexing through its full range, deforming.

Because his tissues are elastic, as the foot leaves the ground the ankle no longer flexes, the range no longer needed. If his ankle were plastic, as the foot left the ground the ankle would remain in the flexed position.

If you are stuck and static stretching isn't working, give yourself permission to try a different way. Often, our preconceived notions of what "should" work limit us from finding what actually works.

But back to lengthening and folding. What do these terms mean and how do they relate to you?

Lengthening and folding: The complementary range pair

To lengthen is to get longer. To extend or stretch. To prolong.

Folding means to bring into a compact form. To make smaller. To use less space.

If you are thinking about lengthening in terms of movement, when you lengthen a limb, what happens to the speed of a movement?

If you don't remember from chapter 2, no worries. The quick recap is this: long is slow, short is fast. So if you need to slow down, you lengthen. If you want to speed up, you fold.

Imagine a diver, performing a tuck jump off the high dive. They jump, tuck, and spin quickly, performing the desired number of rotations before lengthening out. Why do they bother lengthening at all? Because they need to stop the rotation so they can enter the water safely and get the maximum number of aesthetic points. The high-impact collision with the water would cause a rippling of unwanted vibrations; lengthening slows down the collision with the water and enables the diver to have more control over the entry. This control allows the diver to turn unwanted vibrations into wanted vibrations.

Lengthening is simply doing what the diver is doing—spreading out and expanding. You can lengthen your arm overhead or out to the side or behind you. You can lengthen your spine up or your pelvis down. You can lengthen your leg behind you or in front of you or out to the side.

How you lengthen is dependent on an interplay of communication between all of the joints in the limb and torso. Lengthening is not performed in isolation; it's performed in a way that creates connection to the rest of the structure.

Try this: Reach your left arm towards the ceiling. Really imagine your hand is going to touch the ceiling above you. Lower it down. Pause for a moment.

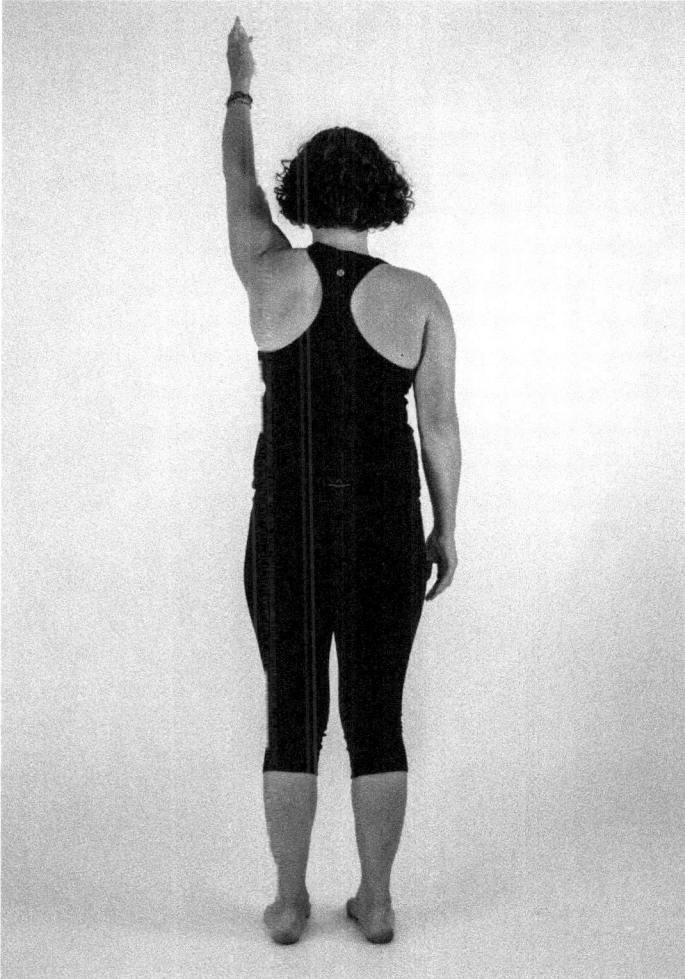

Now, reach your left arm towards the ceiling again, trying to touch the ceiling with your fingers. This time, imagine the left shoulder blade is reaching the arm up. Lower the arm down.

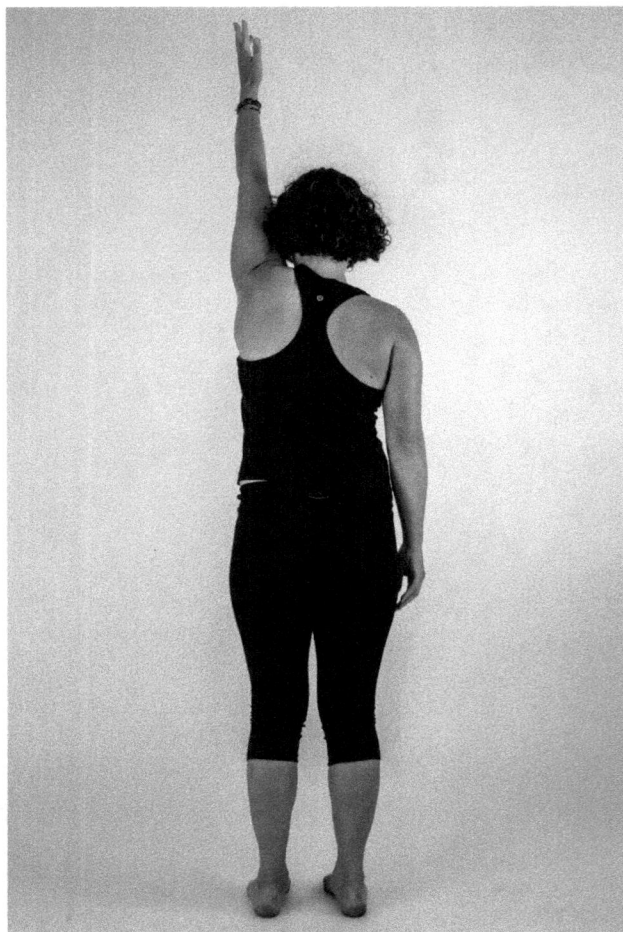

Reach the left arm up towards the ceiling using your left shoulder blade and your left ribs to lengthen the left arm up. Lower the arm down.

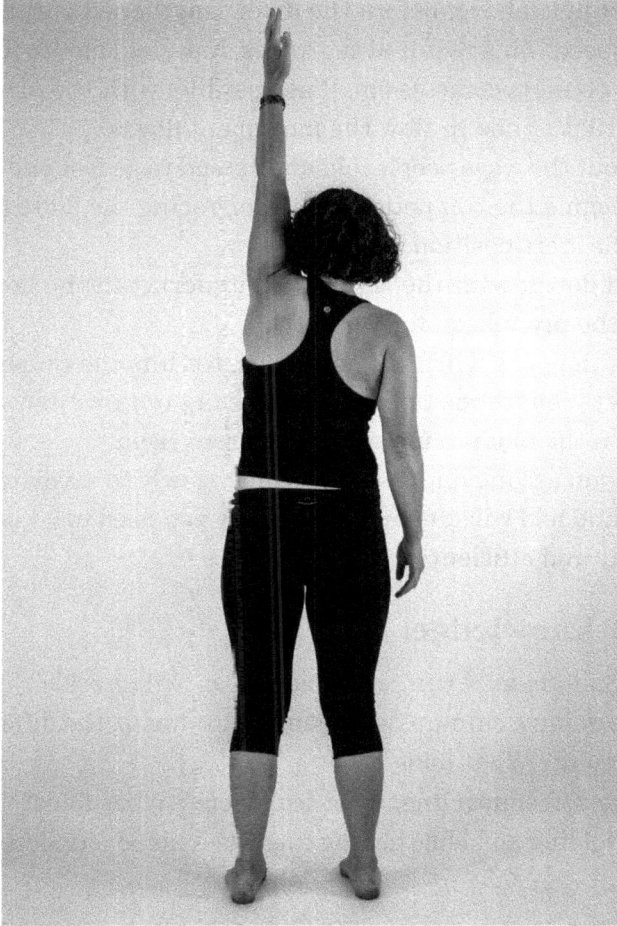

When did you feel like your left arm was the longest and your fingers were able to reach closest to the ceiling? When did it feel like the left fingers were furthest away from the ceiling?

What happens if you try to touch the ceiling with your left palm instead of your left fingers? Does that change things? Does it increase or decrease the connection with your shoulder blade?

In the example above, before the diver lengthened out, they tucked, generating speed. This required the knees, hips, and feet to fold inwards, so the diver could become as small as possible, with the arms touching the body until it's time to slow the movement down.

Think about the ways people fold and extend to go fast and go slow. For instance, imagine the competitive sprinter racing the 200 meter dash—what does the start position look like?

Crouched down, with the legs folded underneath the body in a way that allows the propulsion forward.

And what happens when the same sprinter hits the finish-line tape?

The athlete lengthens up, arms extending out away from the body, slowing down the momentum generated from racing.

Whether you are moving fast to finish or slowly to savor, learning how to lengthen and fold will create the flexibility you need to accomplish most things fluidly and efficiently.

Test your knowledge:

If you go for a four-mile run, what lengthens? What folds?

If you are doing a chin-up, what lengthens during the different phases of the movement? What folds?

If you give someone a hug, what lengthens? What folds?

Ideas for folding and lengthening exercises can be found in the exercise section.

How your foot actually works (and why flattening the foot isn't pronation):

You glimpse a long, bare leg. The calf flexes as a foot steps forward, causing a rippling effect up the leg. The foot is at an angle, the transverse arch supported by high heels, causing a gentle sway as the leg moves by.

Depending on which foot camp you are in, you may have read the above paragraph and thought: High heels. A bare leg. That's sexy. Or, you may have thought: Oh no! Someone needs to tell this person to remove the shoes immediately and begin doing intrinsic foot exercises to save this person's foot from the demise that comes from wearing heels!

Somewhere along the lines of studying feet and learning ways to develop more control in the foot and ankle, some interesting ideas have developed that go against the very architecture of the foot. Wearing heels once in a while, for instance, doesn't necessarily cause permanent foot deformation or osteoarthritis, though it does change how a person walks (Borchgrevink et al., 2016; Barnish & Barnish, 2016; Wiedemeijer & Otten, 2018).

If you have been following along, this should make sense.

Why? Because the foot on the ground can be a class-one or class-two lever. The foot elevated can still be a class-one or class-two lever. What is the difference between an elevated foot and a non-elevated foot?

The amount of range the foot has. When it's elevated, there is less range which means it will go from a class-one to a class-two lever more quickly than if it isn't elevated. This will, in turn, affect how your torso moves over the foot.

Arches and the foot: A review

The foot, if you remember from chapter 4, is a unique structure. It's an architectural masterpiece, with three main arches that bear the weight of the body in a variety of positions. To recap, these three arches are the lateral longitudinal arch, the medial longitudinal arch, and the transverse arch.

If you are thinking, we covered this pretty thoroughly already, bear with me. Understanding how arches work is a really important piece to understanding the body's structure.

Think about the places you have arches. Your feet. Your hands. Your spine. What do these areas have in common?

They support large amounts of weight from various parts of the body regularly. And despite regularly contending with the stress imparted upon them, these areas usually last an entire life time in tact.

This is impressive when you think about it. It's the arched shape of these structures that allows them to withstand compressive load every single day of our lives.

An arch is designed to distribute stress across the structure. An arch bridge, which is literally a bridge that is shaped like an arch underneath, supports different loads by distributing compression across and down the arch. The nature of the arched structure means it's always pushing in on itself (Bridge Masters, 2017).

In our arch bridge example, the bridge has a keystone (a.k.a. capstone). The keystone is the stone at the top of the arch. It plays a critical role in distributing weight down the side supporting blocks—it's the "key" stone because if you remove it, the arch will collapse (Johns, 2010).

What else makes an arch collapse? If the endpoints get further away from each other.

Imagine our hypothetical arched bridge. If you moved one end of the bridge away from the other end of the bridge, the arch would begin to flatten out. If you continued to move the end of the bridge away from the other end, eventually the arch would no longer be an arch and the bridge would collapse.

This is less than ideal (and not exactly possible unless you managed to attain superhero strength), but hopefully you can see how strong an arch actually is.

The foot is built similarly as the arch bridge, complete with keystones that maintain the integrity of the arches and endpoints that aren't designed to move far away from each other (Samim et al., 2016; Gwani et al., 2017).

Before we move on, ask yourself this: do you want the arch bridge to collapse a little bit every time you drive over it?

I don't like my bridges collapsing every time I put weight on them, even if it's just a little bit.

Which brings us to the question of what allows movement in the foot. Since the three arches of the foot are designed to work together to provide an integrated system of three bridges to support you as you move throughout the world, the bones in these metaphorical bridges withstand compressive forces not by collapsing, but by resisting a change in shape. Movement, then, occurs because of dynamic ankle flexion, which you learned about in chapter 4. The shin pitches forward, providing compression to the subtalar joint (a fancy name for the area in front of the ankle-joint complex where movement happens). And when the shin pitches forward, the foot pitches forward as well.

This can be a weird thing to imagine initially, but when the foot pitches forward, it isn't like the foot leaves the ground and suddenly shifts position in space. Rather, the place where the shin attaches (the ankle) causes the weight to shift towards the middle and front of the foot. The heel responds by leaving the ground.

This happens because the calcaneus rolls; everything else responds by folding and lengthening (Elftman, 1969).

The pitch, yaw, and roll of the foot are all detected at the transverse arch. How you move over the foot (and how strong the foot feels) is determined by what the transverse arch senses.

Adarian put it this way, "Arches are the foundation of movement from bottom to top. Ankle flexion is the articulation."

Another way to think of this is that arches create the foundation on which movement can occur. The foot detects weight shift. This creates sensory input in the ankle joint through pitch and roll, which the CNS uses to determine the subsequent movement.

If the arches support you, is it necessary to do foot exercises? And if the sensory input in the ankle joint is critical for the CNS, what sensory input are foot exercises providing to enhance dynamic, every day foot and ankle function?

If foot exercises are your thing, by all means keep doing them. But they aren't going to make your foot function better. If you are searching for better foot control, learn to understand your arches by using the mapping exercises in the next section and practice how to flex your ankle. Use your arches as arches and find dynamic movement through the ankle for a foot that can withstand stress and generate movement.

Here's the thing about the ankle—it will only flex during dynamic situations. You can think of dynamic movement as movement that happens when you are moving your body weight over your foot in some way.

What does that mean for things like calf raises? While a standing calf raise can be useful to help someone feel the shift in weight from the heels to the balls of the feet, they don't actually work the ankle in a dynamic range of motion. What this means is when you are actually moving through space, the demands of the range of motion at the ankle joint are higher than when you are standing at a wall lifting your heels.

Again, as we have said repeatedly, if you like doing calf raises, do calf raises, but if you want to challenge the ankle and foot in a way that mimics the demands they need for everyday life, ankle and foot training needs to be approached in a more dynamic way.

One of the amazing things about the human body during movement is its ability to withstand various stresses. The foot and ankle withstand the stress of gravity and the weight shift that occurs during movement through the formation of arches and the corresponding deformation that occurs at the ankle. When you understand the range at the ankle and the corresponding movement at the foot through the lens of pitch, yaw, and roll, it becomes easier to see how to create strong, stable feet and ankles in a way that transfers to the things you do during your everyday life, whether that's chase your children, run six miles, or play basketball.

Your core and rotation:

The curve of the low back as the hips move. The shape of the waist as the arms reach. The change in muscle tone of the belly as you lie down and sit up.

The spine (which is twenty-four joints) runs from your head to your pelvis, like the foot, and consists of three arches. These arches are different from the foot in a number of ways—not only are they longer, but they run vertically rather than horizontally. Instead of an arch bridge that you move across, the spine is a vertical structure designed to be stressed in a variety of positions. This creates strain throughout the spine but, because the spine is comprised of arches, the strain is dispersed across the structure.

If you are standing and I place my hands on your shoulders and press downward, you stay upright, with minimal movement down. This is like walking over the bridge and not having it dip downward with each step. The compression is distributed over the arches, allowing the spine to remain intact (Galbusera & Bassani, 2019).

The muscles of the spine are designed to allow a lot of forces to be placed upon it in a variety of ways. The strongest muscles of the back run along the spinal column, allowing the spine to bend. The bend of the spine is supported by your six-pack muscle, which has a long-lever arm and supports the weight of the torso. And then, of course, there are muscles that allow the spine to laterally flex and rotate (Vasavada et al., 2010).

Think of the sit-up, a traditional exercise that is currently labeled as "bad" by a lot of people in the fitness industry even though you sit-up whenever you transition from lying down to upright. The sitting up portion of the sit-up is actually a good thing—it's a movement you perform regularly and one that your spine is designed to handle well.

The potential problem with the sit-up comes when you keep the spine rounded. As you bend back, your spine becomes a suspension bridge. The weight of the head creates a backwards load far away from the fulcrum (which is the hips). How you present the load or stress is dependent on the position of the spine as you lower down and come up.

Imagine the person with a bulging six-pack. While this may be considered aesthetically pleasing for some, it's not a good thing for the spine. A bulging six-pack will alter the way the spine handles strain, which ultimately alters how you move.

This ability of the spine to move and respond as you move and respond, all while resisting downward compression, is kind of incredible when you think about it. In fact, while you are thinking about it, imagine this: you pick up a barbell that weighs more than you. Your spine doesn't buckle under the load. Instead, it adjusts position so that it doesn't buckle, because the sensory input from the load and your joints determines how you pick up the barbell. You set it down and repeat (or not, depending on whether you feel like lifting a barbell repeatedly).

This is kind of amazing. Almost as amazing as the contortionist, who, from a standing position, bends backwards until their elbows are on the floor, smiling the entire time. They reverse out of it, as though nothing has happened.

Not everyone wants to be able to withstand the compressive force of a barbell, and the vast majority of us aren't doing extreme backbends for fun. But most of us are unloading the dishwasher, putting clothes away on the top shelf, and dragging the garbage cans out to the curb. We are using our spines in a dynamic way every single day.

Before we go on, yes, low back pain happens. So do ankle sprains. And meniscus tears. And shoulder pain. But those things aren't the point of this book, and if you are experiencing low back pain (or any of the other conditions I just rattled off), please go see your medical provider for care.

The point is, you are designed to move a lot of different ways. That includes your spine.

The myth of core strengthening and core stability:

What does it mean for something to be stable? Merriam-Webster's Collegiate Dictionary (n.d.) defines stability as, "the quality, state, or degree of being stable. The strength to stand or endure." Something that is stable is something that is designed to return to its original condition when disturbed from a state of equilibrium.

Another way to think of stability is that it's a quality related to homeostasis. There is balance between how the structures related to the spine allow movement, just like there is an inherent balance in your internal landscape. You can get knocked off-center or you can purposefully move from center and return to a place where you feel safe and secure, not wobbly or unsure.

Remember, too, that you are composed of simple machines called levers that produce movement. How you use these levers is determined by sensory input. If you believe that you are weak, that is an input because your thoughts are an input.

This leads us to core strengthening and core stability. If you are cleared for exercise by your physical therapist or doctor and you want to get stronger, do you need core specific exercises to protect your low back?

In athletes, the answer appears to be inconclusive at best (Wirth et al., 2017). Core-stability exercises often fall into the following categories: antirotation exercises, anti-extension exercises, and antiflexion exercises.

Remember that levers work by an initiation of rotation. This causes a sequential domino effect, allowing movement to occur. So is training the core in a way that eliminates using the lever arms an effective path for movement freedom?

And if it isn't, what should you do instead?

If the goal is to create a strong, healthy spine, doing some sort of back-bend for spine health will make you (and your spine) more adaptable. It's an important part of "core" training, and if you are curious about ideas on how to do it, there are exercises in the next section that focus on just that.

If your goal is to do a cool acrobatics trick, figure out the levers involved. Train the different pieces. Put the pieces together. The core will become strong in the way it needs to become stronger.

If you are working on improving your sprinting speed, make your lever arms work for you. Practice sprinting while focusing on timing, sequencing, and coordination. Your core will figure out how to support you.

Assess the levers. Train the levers. What are you trying to do? If your goal is a specific skill, train the skill while paying attention to how you use the levers. The core musculature will adapt accordingly.

And if you love doing core-stability exercises and antirotation exercises, by all means, keep doing them. But if your goal is to find a sense of elation through moving in a way that is dynamic and powerful, embrace rotation and the freedom that comes when you begin to self organize in a way that takes advantage of input in the form of pressure and the lever arms that produce movement. You are capable of so much more than you think—it's just a matter of learning how to use what you have.

Train different. Train fast. Train faster.

THE EXERCISES

O kay, you made it through the how: how things work when you exercise, perform an athletic skill, or move. The concepts remain the same regardless of what you are doing; what changes is the what. And now that you are armed with the knowledge about *how* you can ask yourself if *what* you are doing supports *why* you are doing it.

The exercises that follow are divided into three categories: range, compression, and strength. Range refers to exercises that develop range. Compression refers to exercises the emphasize compression. Strength refers to exercises that develop strength. (We like to keep things simple.) Some exercises fall into multiple categories.

The sample program at the end of the section provides an idea for how the exercises can be used to create a general exercise program that addresses both range and strength, but it's just an idea. If you are trying to get faster at a specific sport, you might need more strength and less range, or if you are trying to improve your range of motion so you can throw faster or kick your leg up and over a fence, you might need more range.

The point is, use the exercises and/or suggested program to enhance an aspect of your life in some way, whether it's to run faster, garden more efficiently, or flow more easily. Once you have played with the exercises for a while, don't be afraid to take the concepts and apply them to other exercises, or maybe even invent your own exercises. What matters is applying the concepts you have already learned. If you adhere to the underlying principles discussed in the previous pages, you can find ways to move that will achieve whatever it is that you want to achieve. So go and enjoy the process.

The exercises:

Under each exercise you will see a line devoted to its purpose. This briefly describes whether the exercise is a range exercise, a strength exercise, or something else. The different exercise categories and their descriptions can be found below.

Range exercises:

Range exercises explore how far the *effort* moves. If I reach my arm overhead and my arm stops before it's pointing up towards the ceiling, the effort is when my arm stops moving. If I reach through my shoulder blade as I reach up towards the ceiling and my arm reaches more towards the ceiling, my range (and therefore my effort) will be greater.

Compression exercises:

Compression exercises are designed to create pressure in joints. Remember that pressure is a way to improve body mapping, improve the system's sense of safety, and produce the desired movement.

Strength exercises:

These exercises are designed to increase strength. This means range will be shorter, but effort will be higher.

Exercise 1: Torso Lengthening

Purpose: range through torso
This exercise comes in three different vartiations:

Variation A:

- Standing, feet are wherever

- Slight squat if desired (progression)

- Reach arms forward, move arms overhead and continue reaching

Key points: pull from side of torso to hip
Things to watch for: shoulder tightening

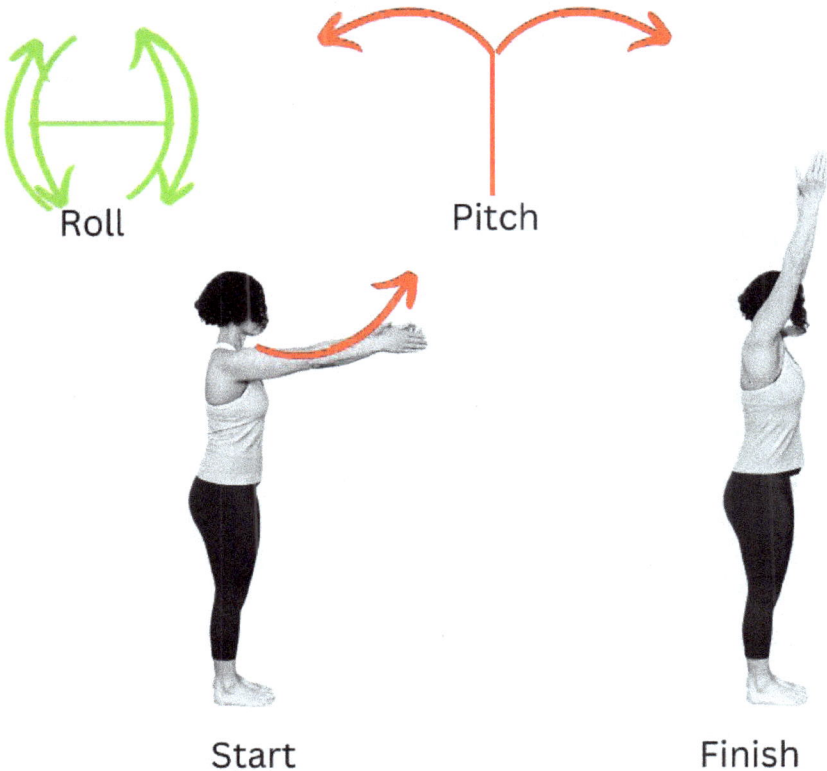

Roll

Pitch

Start

Finish

Variation B:

- Standing, feet are wherever
- Slight squat if desired (progression)
- Reach elbows forward and up, move elbows overhead and continue reaching

Key points: pull from side of torso to hip
Things to watch for: shoulder tightening

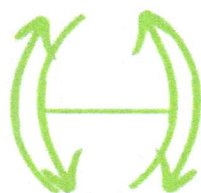
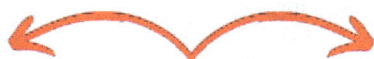
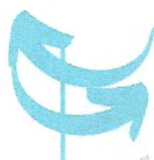

Roll   Pitch   Yaw

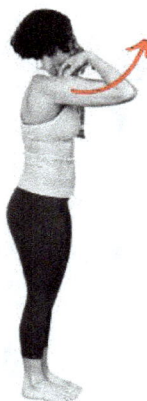
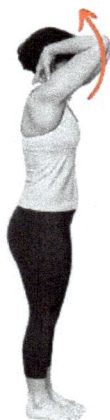
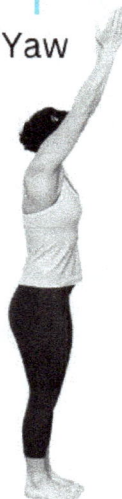

Start   Middle   Finish

Variation C:

- Standing, feet are wherever
- Slight squat if desired (progression)
- Reach arms back, palms reaching as though to grab something
- Keep reaching as they move overhead and forward
- Feel torso respond at the top of the movement

Key points: lead with the palm, not the fingers
Things to watch for: don't shrug up or cave the chest

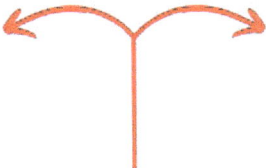

Pitch

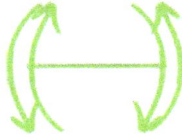

Roll

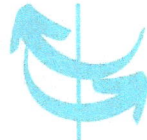

Yaw

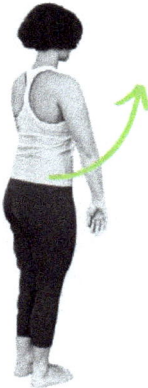

Start

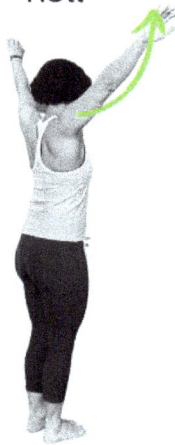

Middle

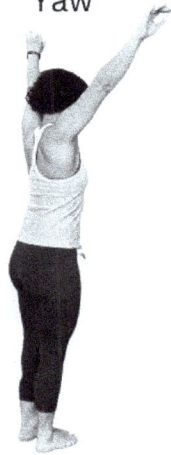

Finish

Exercise 2: Sitting in the Bucket

Purpose: strength through legs

- Standing, feet are wherever (Have videos)
- Reach butt cheeks back, pitch torso forward

Key points: actively reach palms forward, sit back and let joints work their magic

Things to watch for: not a squat, not a hinge, make sure you allow the knees to bend

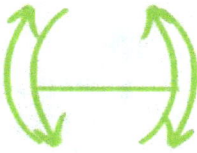

Roll

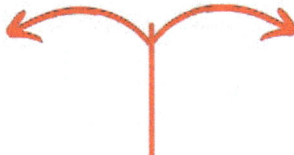

Pitch

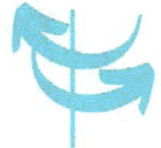

Yaw

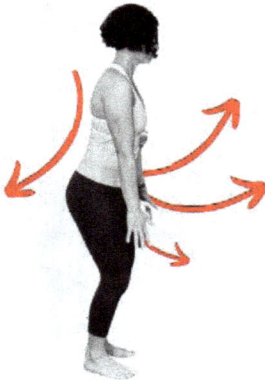

Start

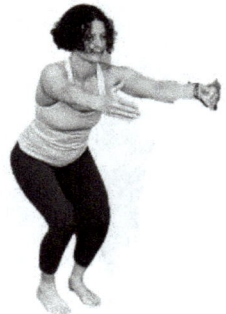

Finish

Exercise 3: Arm Lengthening While Sitting in the Bucket

Purpose: strength and range through arms and legs

- Standing, feet are wherever
- Reach butt cheeks back, pitch torso forward, reach palms forward and up

Key points: actively reach palms forward, let joints work their magic

Things to watch for: not a squat, not a hinge, make sure you allow the knees to bend

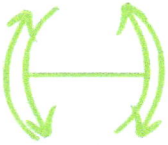
Roll

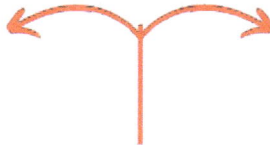
Pitch

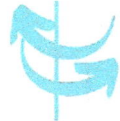
Yaw

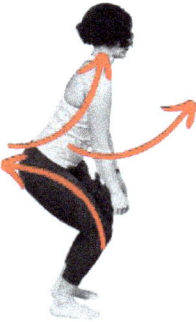
Start

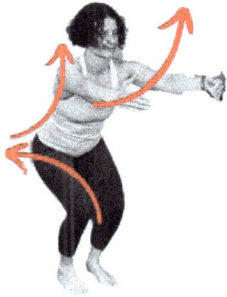
Middle

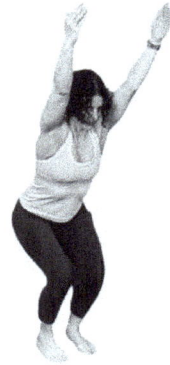
Finish

Exercise 4: Pinky Toe and Quad Squats

Purpose: strengthening

This exercise comes in two different variations:

Variation A:

- Standing, feet are wherever (Have videos)
- Push your pinky toe down as you push down on one leg

Key points: avoid the knee

Things to watch for: don't do a pistol squat or a squat where you emphasize keeping the heel down while the other leg extends in front of you.

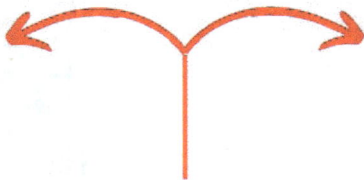
Pitch

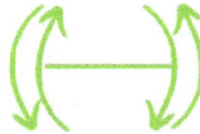
Roll

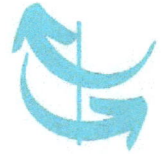
Yaw

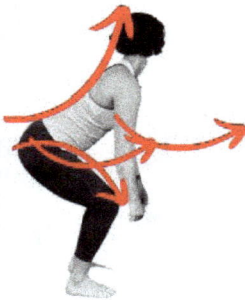
Start

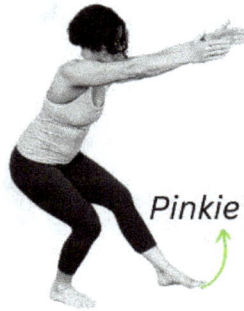
Pinkie toe rolls

Finish

Variation B:

Purpose: Compression leg in lever-two mode

- Standing, reach the pinky toe long, lift the other leg up
- Shift the weight to the pinky toe, lift the other leg up behind you, front knee and hip will flex naturally.

Key points: reach as far back as you can with the free leg, back leg serves as anchor

Things to watch for: don't initially tense anything, don't turn into a single-leg dead lift

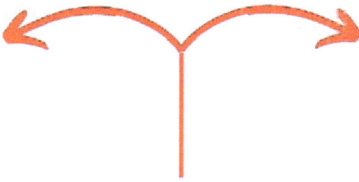

Pitch

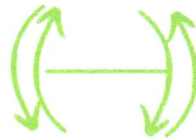

Roll

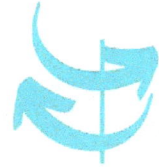

Yaw

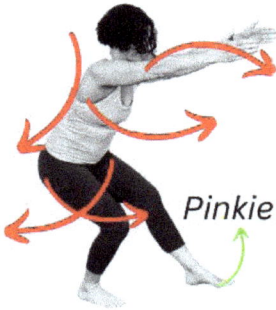

Pinkie toe rolls

Start

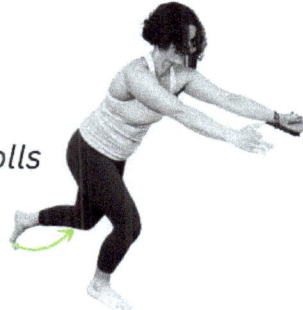

Pinkie toe rolls

Finish

Exercise 5: Oblique Compression

Purpose: compression

- Standing, feet are wherever
- Place hands on belly and move down and in

Key points: make sure you go down, not forward or pulling in the transverse abdominis

Things to watch for: don't tuck your pelvis, don't brace your abdomen

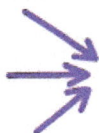

Compression

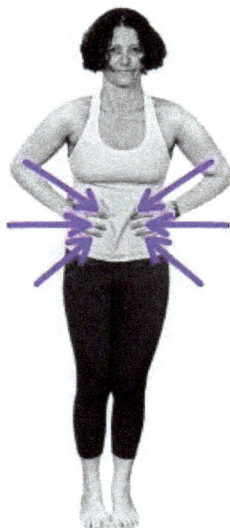

Exercise 6: Arch Squat

Purpose: strength through legs and feet (can also be compression, can be done fast or slow)

- Standing, weight on one foot
- Set transverse arch, pull heel toward ball of the foot (like an inchworm), butt goes straight toward heel, creating a squat

Key points: all of the arches are used

Things to watch for: don't perform the movement by shortening the foot, heel stays down

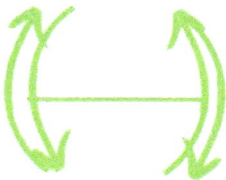

Roll

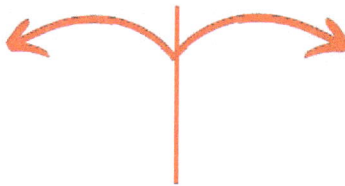

Pitch

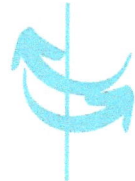

Yaw

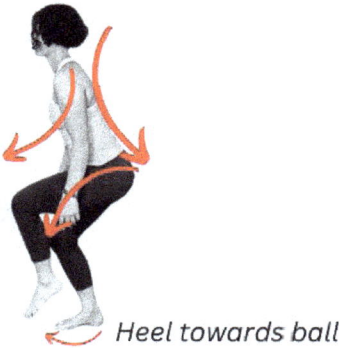

Heel towards ball

Start

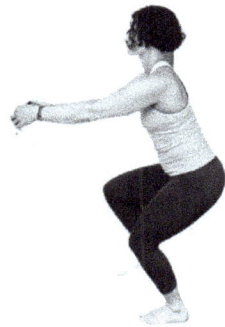

Finish

Exercise 7: Standing Hip Thrust

Purpose: range

This exercise comes in two different variations:

Variation A:

- Standing, feet are wherever
- Set pinky toes and transverse arch, lift heels, drive butt straight down which sends you forward

Key points: the further butt goes down, the further hips go forward

Things to watch for: not a Sissy squat

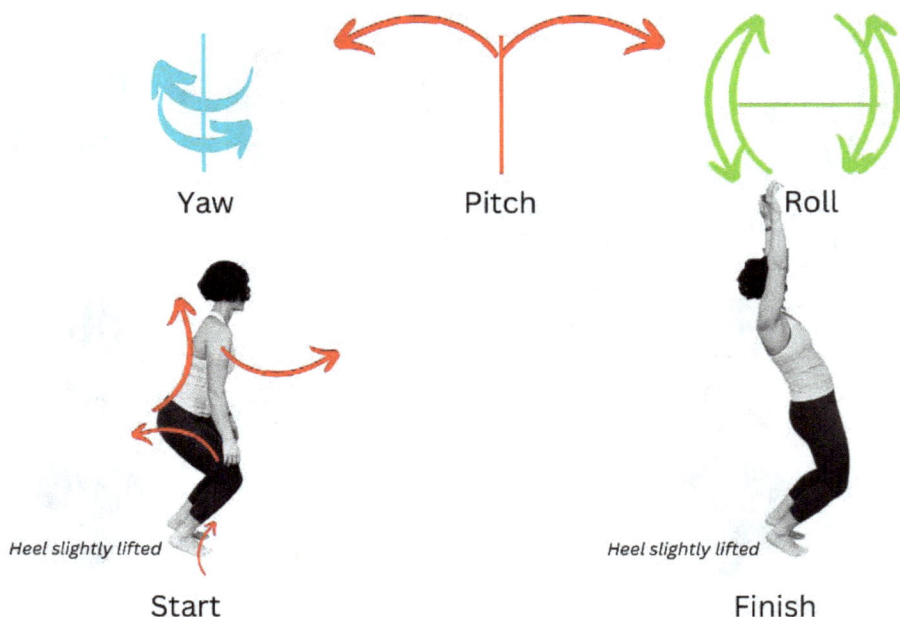

Yaw   Pitch   Roll

Heel slightly lifted   *Heel slightly lifted*

Start   Finish

Variation B:

Stand on one leg, apply same points

Key points: the further butt goes down, the further hips go forward

Things to watch for: not a Sissy squat

Exercise 8: Robot Walk

Purpose: body mapping of obliques, scapula, from head to toe

- Standing, transfer weight to one foot
- Set transverse arch, set gastrocnemius
- Same side oblique as weighted foot reaches back and around, allowing you to take a step

Key points: same side oblique has to reach back and around, gastrocnemius has to be engaged

Things to watch for: hip doesn't do the movement, ipsilateral movement, not contralateral

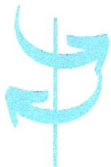
Yaw

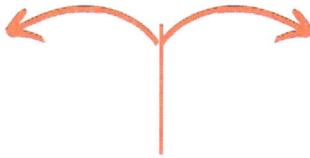
Pitch

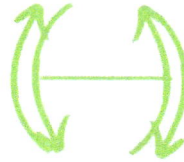
Roll

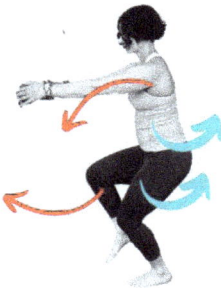
Start

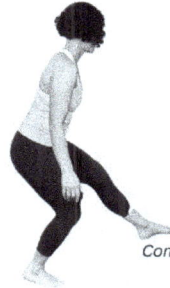

Complete by taking a step

Finish

Exercise 9: Rapid Eccentric

Purpose: extension range (fast)

- Standing, start on one leg
- Heel and pinky toe of unweighted leg reach towards the ground at the exact same time

Key points: reach for the ground like someone is reaching the foot towards the ground, fast, let the joint stop you

Things to watch for: not a kick

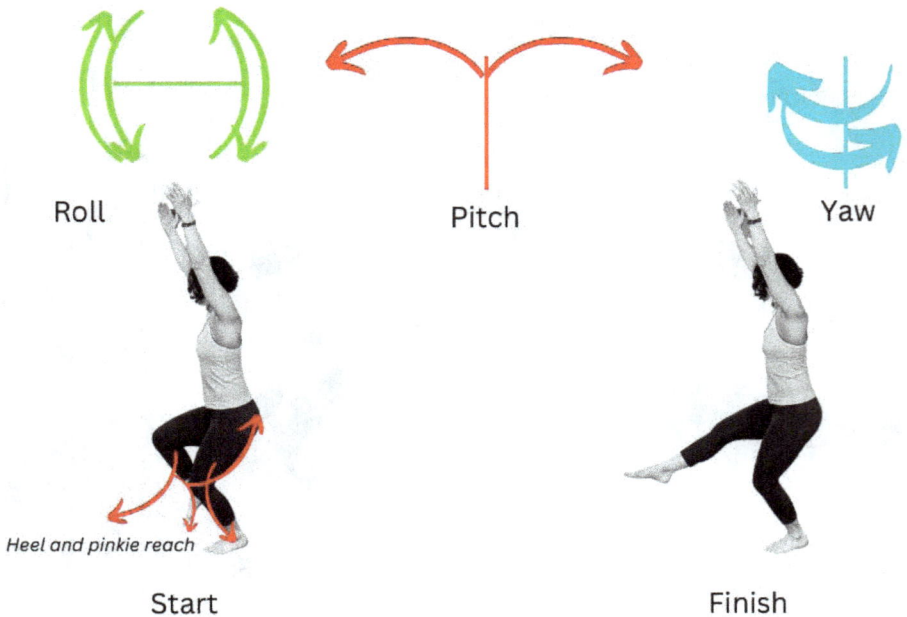

Roll

Pitch

Yaw

Heel and pinkie reach

Start

Finish

Exercise 10: Walking Torso Flex

Purpose: strength and speed

- Stand on one leg
- Using hip flexor and using only unweighted leg, pull entire body forward
- Move forward, one step at a time

Key points: plantar flexion
Things to watch for: don't sit back on it, not a hinge

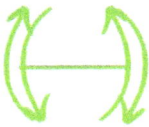

Roll

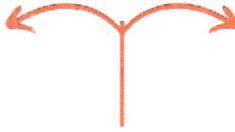

Pitch

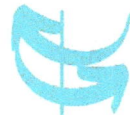

Yaw

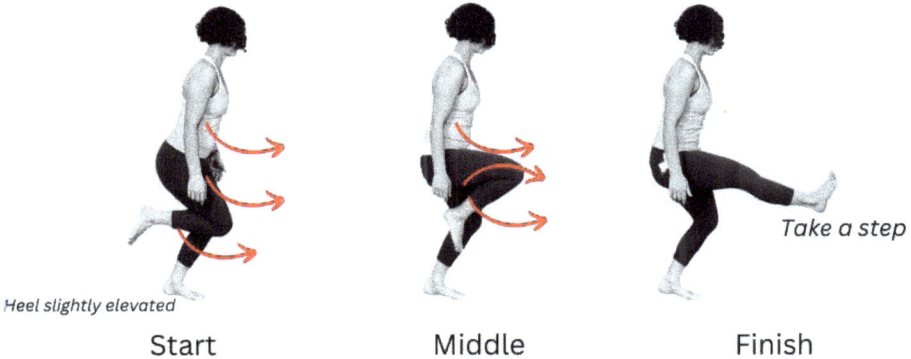

Heel slightly elevated

Start

Middle

Take a step

Finish

Exercise 11: Arm Wave for Scapula

Purpose: range

- Standing
- In sequence, start wave at shoulder blade and then, shoulder, elbow, wrist

Key points: any direction works
Things to watch for: don't skip any joints

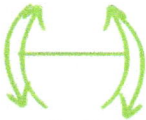

Roll

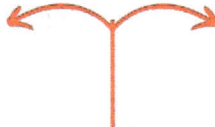

Pitch

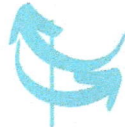

Yaw

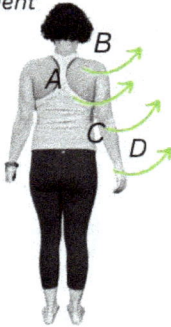

Start

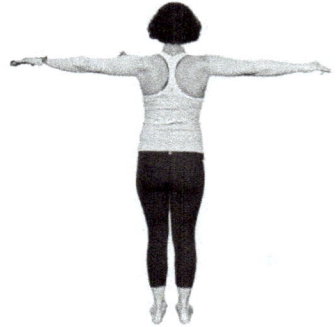

Finish

Exercise 12: Palm and Foot Splay

Purpose: body mapping/range

- Standing, palms splay, transverse arches splay
- Palms rotate up, feet rotate out

Key points: pinky finger will drop down if transverse arch splays; if it doesn't splay, it will flare

Things to watch for: don't splay the fingers, don't splay the toes, don't grip the ground with the toes

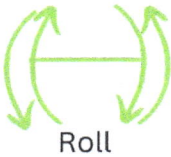
Roll

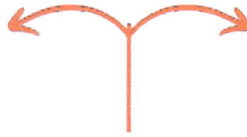
Pitch

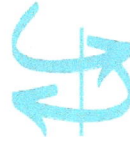
Yaw

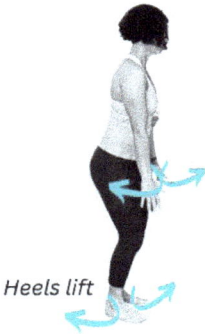
Heels lift
Start

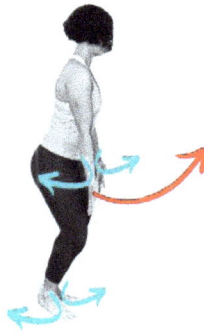
Middle

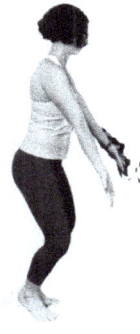
Finish

Exercise 13: Glute Lift

Purpose: range, range with hip extension
This exercise comes in two different variations:

Variation A: extended

- Standing on one leg, other leg is behind
- Extended leg reaches back first, up second

Key points: keep the back leg straight as you lengthen
Things to watch for: don't rotate, don't reach up first, don't curl the heel up

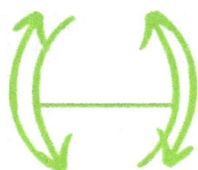

Roll

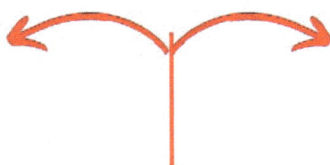

Pitch

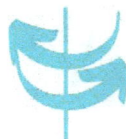

Yaw

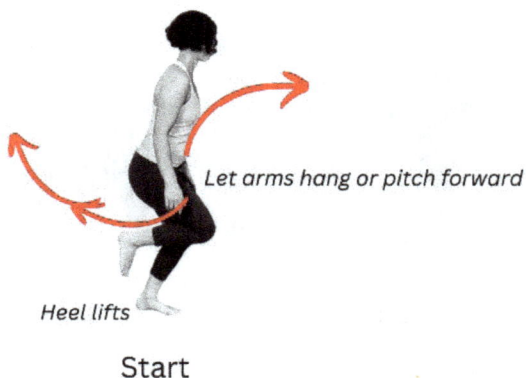

Let arms hang or pitch forward

Heel lifts

Start

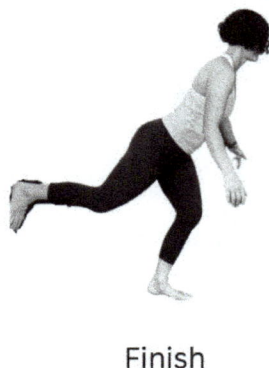

Finish

Variation B: bent knee

- Standing on one leg, other leg is behind
- Extended leg reaches back first, up second

Key points: keep the back leg straight as you lengthen

Things to watch for: don't rotate, don't reach up first, don't curl the heel up

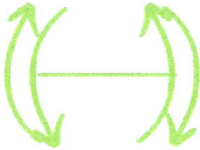

Roll

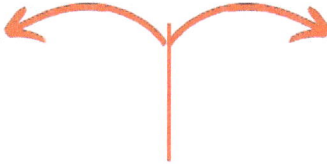

Pitch

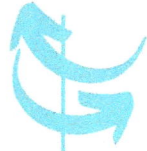

Yaw

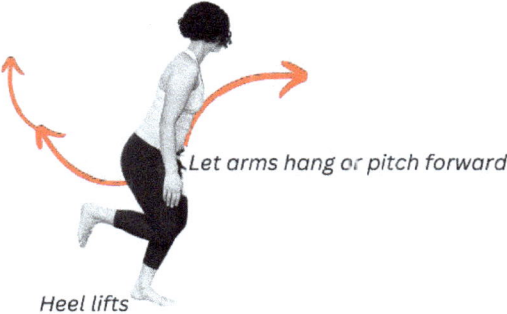

Let arms hang or pitch forward

Heel lifts

Start

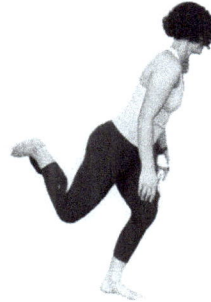

Finish

Exercise 14: Lean Back to Tall

Purpose: range, class-two lever

- Standing
- Lean back, heels up, knees bent
- Straighten knee and move back, heels stay where they are

Key points: alignment comes from knees, not from everything straightening up

Things to watch for: don't press from the ankle up

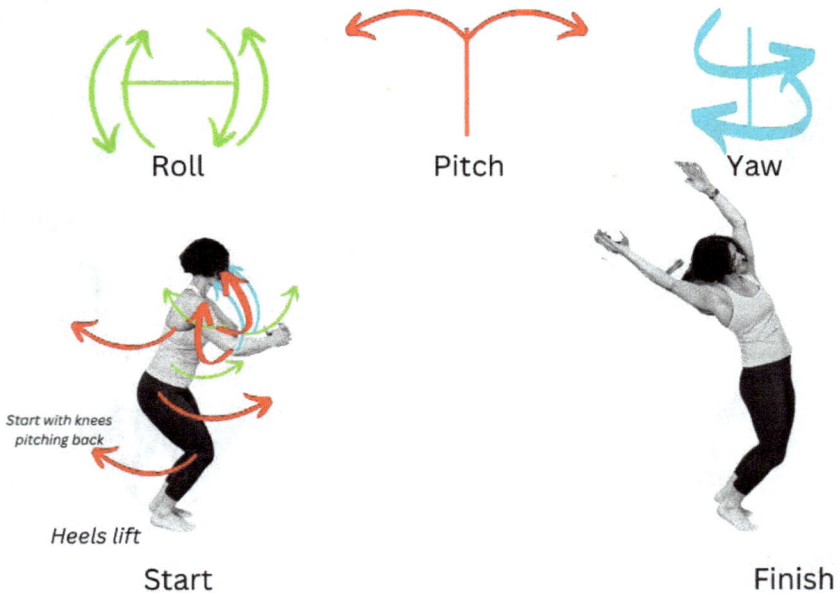

Roll

Pitch

Yaw

Start with knees
pitching back

Heels lift

Start

Finish

Exercise 15: Press Up from Floor

Purpose: strength

- Seated in long sit, hands by your sides or on yoga blocks
- Use hip flexors to pull lower body into upper body

Key points: create balance between upper and lower body (happens when you use hip flexors)

Things to watch for: use hip flexors, not triceps

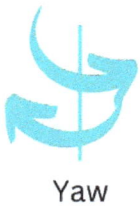

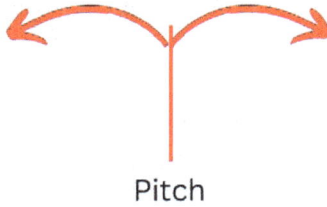

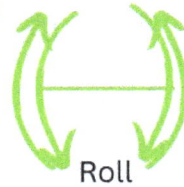

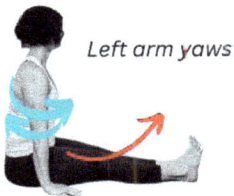

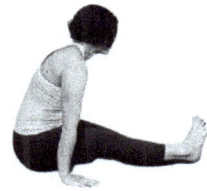

Yaw   Pitch   Roll

Left arm yaws

Start   Finish

Exercise 16: Self Lever

Purpose: range and balance

This exercise comes in two different variations:

Variation A: leg extended

- Standing, squat down a little bit on one one leg, other leg is in front

- Extended leg reaches up

- When you run out of range, torso responds and leans back

Key points: let torso respond

Things to watch for: don't stand flat-footed (standing leg heel can come up), don't arch your back, not a hinge

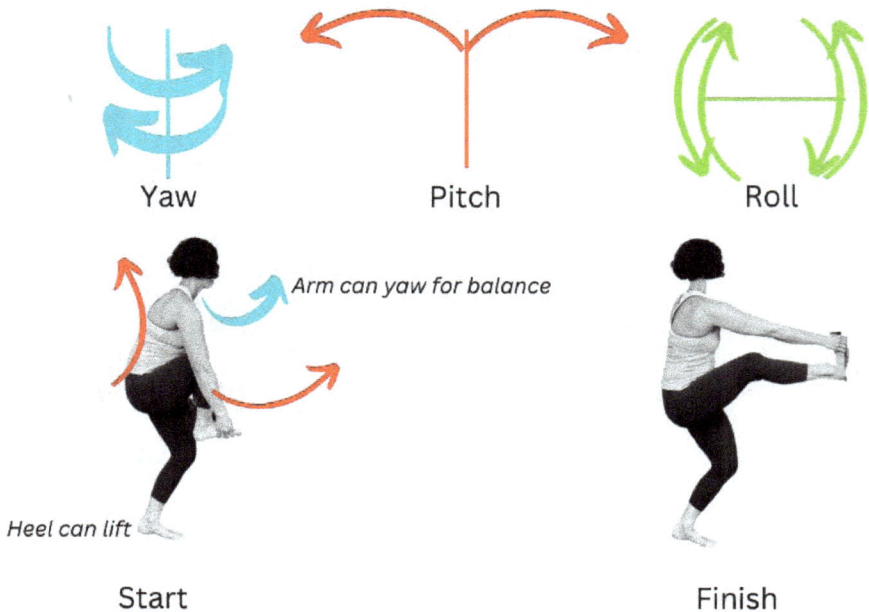

Yaw   Pitch   Roll

Arm can yaw for balance

Heel can lift

Start   Finish

Variation B: Leg extended hold foot

Purpose: range

- Standing, squat down a little bit on one one leg, other leg is in front
- Hold foot with same side of hand
- Extended leg reaches up
- When you run out of range, torso responds and leans back

Key points: let torso respond

Things to watch for: don't stand flat-footed (standing leg heel can come up), don't arch your back, not a hinge

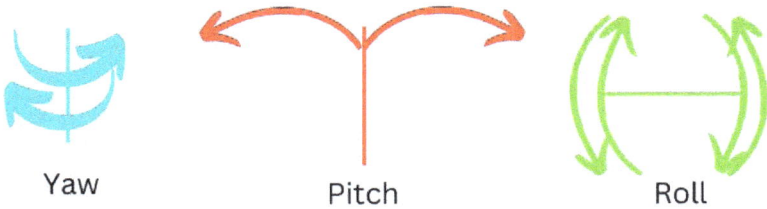

Yaw   Pitch   Roll

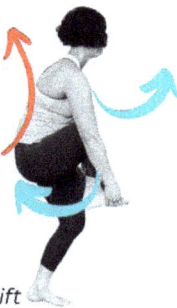

Heel can lift

Start

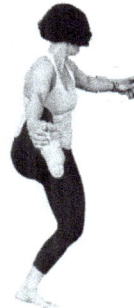

Finish

Exercise 17: Modified Knee Hugger

Purpose: range

- Standing, squat down a little bit on one leg, hug other knee in front of you
- Lean torso back
- Heel comes off ground

Key points: let torso respond

Things to watch for: don't stand flat-footed (standing leg heel can come up), don't arch your back, not a hinge

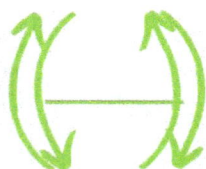

Roll

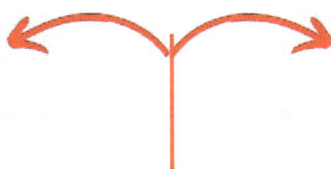

Pitch

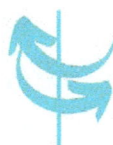

Yaw

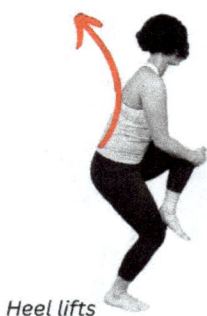

Heel lifts

Start

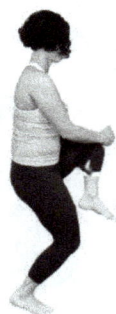

Finish

Exercise 18: Single Leg Rotation

Purpose: range

- Standing, squat down, heels come up
- Lift one leg with bent knee
- Rotate unweighted leg in a variety of directions

Key points: have fun, go with the flow

Things to watch for: not letting the heel come up, externally rotating the leg but not letting the torso respond

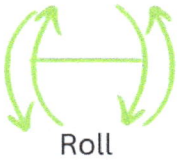

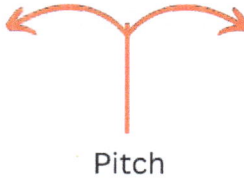

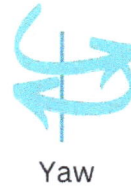

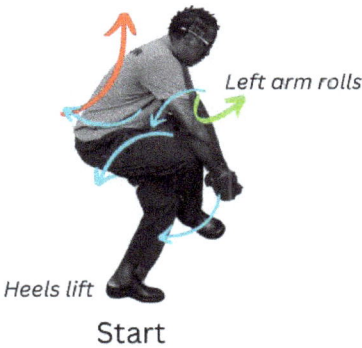

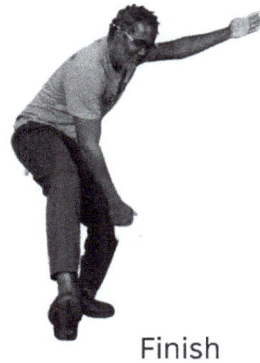

Roll   Pitch   Yaw

Left arm rolls

Heels lift

Start   Finish

IN CONCLUSION

YOU'RE JUST GETTING STARTED

A Google search brings up elation defined as "great happiness and exhilaration." It is the feeling you had as a child when you climbed to the top of the stairs for the first time without help, or when you swung across the monkey bars, skipping a bar occasionally to see how fast you could go.

Movement is a source of elation in a number of ways. It's the thing that allows you to breathe, make food, have sex, run a marathon, or dance. Understanding how you move creates a deeper connection to the act of moving. Moving isn't something to fear; it's something to embrace becase it means you are alive.

We wrote this book to give you an opportunity to explore what it means to move. You produce movement through a series of simple machines called levers; these levers can create an infinite number of movements, all based on sensory input.

We hope that by thinking about these concepts, you become curious about moving in a way that brings a sense of exultation and empowerment. The innate intelligence of the body you inhabit enables you to shift how you move by changing the application of resistance or stress. This changes the strain, which changes the resulting action.

The action, of course, is the movement.

Is it really that simple, you may be wondering? Give it a try. See what happens.

TYPES OF LEVERS

A lever is a simple machine that is made up of a lever arm and a fulcrum. In the human body, the rigid beam is analogous to a bone and the fulcrum can be thought of as a joint. For instance, if your foot is on the floor and you bend your knee, you have two fulcrums: the ankle and the hip The thigh and the shin are the lever arms.

If your foot is off the ground and you bend your knee, the knee is the fulcrum and the lever arm is the shin.

Why? Because the anchor points are different in the two scenarios. When the anchor point shifts, the lever arms shift.

In order for movement to occur, effort must overcome resistance. Where the resistance is located on the lever will impact how much effort is needed to overcome the resistance.

In the example of the knee joint, when the foot is on the ground the effort is applied at the hips by the thigh muscles and at the ankle by the calf muscles. The resistance is bidirectional. Gravity pulls you down into the ground as you work to resist gravity by pressing your foot into the ground. When the effort exerted by the thigh and calf muscles overcomes the resistance, the thigh and the lower legs rotate away from each other as the leg straightens. This rotation occurs at the fulcrum points, which are the hip and ankle. The knee simply responds.

How do you impact whether it takes a lot of effort or a little effort to do this?

You can add external resistance so there's more "you" pressing into the ground or you can change the position of the torso. This will change how much resistance the foot is contending with, which will affect how much resistance you have to overcome to stand back up.

Examples include squatting with weight, squatting with the torso forward, squatting with the torso vertical, or squatting with the torso behind the hips (e.g., a Sissy squat).

For the record, we are fully aware the lever arm changes when you are doing a Sissy squat versus when you are doing a regular squat, and that there is no hip flexion.

What about when the foot is off the ground? How does movement work in that situation?

When the foot is off the ground, the load becomes the foot. The effort comes from the muscles that straighten and bend the knee.

How can you change the amount of effort needed?

You can add external load around the ankle (if you add it around the foot, you are adding it an extra lever—the ankle joint). Or you can change the position of the foot relative to the knee. If the foot is in front of the knee as you straighten and bend the knee, it will feel different than if the foot is behind the knee as you straighten and bend the knee. The different positions will require different degrees of effort from the muscles in the front and back of the thigh to overcome the load of the foot.

Torque:

In order for a lever to work, torque is required. Torque is the amount of force needed to create rotation around the axis. When the knee bends with the foot off the ground, there is a certain amount of force the hamstring muscle must exert for the shin to rotate around the knee.

You can think of torque as the thing that gets a wheel turning. When a bike isn't moving, it takes more effort to get the wheels to spin than when the bike is already moving. How much torque is required to perform a movement depends on whether you are starting from a complete standstill or if you are already in motion.

How much load a lever can move depends on the location of the effort, the load, and the fulcrum. This is also called mechanical advantage.

For instance, you can bend the knee with the leg straight out in front of you. You can bend the knee with the leg behind you. You can bend the knee with the leg out to the side of you. You can bend the knee with the foot on the ground or the foot off the ground. All of these conditions alter the position of the muscle that bends the knee, which means the location of the effort changes. This affects how much effort is required to bend the knee. The farther the effort is away from the axis of rotation or fulcrum, the easier it is to move the load. This means it's actually easier to bend the knee when the leg is fully extended than when it is already partially bent and you are trying to bend it more.

Class-one levers:

A class-one lever can be thought of as a teeter-totter. The fulcrum (remember, this is the axis of rotation), is located between the load and the effort.

In the body, the place where your skull meets your spine is a class-one lever. The skull is the lever arm. The fulcrum is the atlanto-occipital joint. The effort is the neck muscles. This arrangement allows the head to nod up and down.

Class-one levers also often occur when there is an external load being moved. When you clean a barbell, for example, the torso becomes the lever arm, pulling the weight from the ground up into a rack position. When you hip thrust, the torso is the lever arm, allowing the weight on the hips to move towards the floor and away from the floor.

Class-one levers slow things down by either multiplying the speed of muscle movements in exchange for decreased strength or multiplying the force of muscle in exchange for decreased speed. The foot, for instance, can act as a class-one lever, slowing things down as the body passes over it.

Class-two levers:

A class-two lever resembles what happens when you use a wheelbarrow. The reason you are able to move heavy loads using a wheelbarrow is because of the way the lever is arranged. The fulcrum is the wheel and is at the end of the lever. The load is the barrow and is somewhere between the effort and the fulcrum.

Imagine a wheelbarrow that is filled with dirt. The dirt is heavy. It represents the load. The wheel is on one side of the load. In order to lift the dirt, you exert effort on the handle, which is on the other side of the load. The long handle is the lever arm.

In the body, a class-two lever occurs at the ankle joint when you stand on your tiptoes. The fulcrum is at the toe joints. The load is your body weight, and the effort is the muscular contraction of the calf muscles. This arrangement allows for a lot of mechanical advantage, which is why such a small area (the ball of the foot) can easily lift up something heavy, like the weight of the body.

Class-three levers:

In a class-three lever, the load is at one end, the fulcrum is at the other, and the effort is in the middle. A pair of tweezers is an example of a class-three lever. The fulcrum is at one end of the tweezers. The load is located at the other. In other to grab the load, the effort is applied to the middle of the tweezers.

Most of the levers in the body without external resistance are class-three levers. When you bend your knee with your foot off the ground, the knee is the fulcrum. The load is the lower leg. The hamstring muscle provides the effort to move the lower leg. Class-three levers have less mechanical advantage than the other two types of levers, so they are less good at moving heavy things, but they excel at generating speed. Most of the joints in the human body are class-three levers. This means the human body is designed for speed. As soon as you add external resistance, the lever arm changes because load is suddenly placed outside the body. The lever converts to a class-one lever, slowing things down.

REFERENCES

Chapter 1:

1. Bacabac R.G., Smit T.H., Van Loon J.J.W.A., Doulabi B.Z., Helder M., & Klein-Nulend J. (2006). Bone cell responses to high-frequency vibration stress: Does the nucleus oscillate within the cytoplasm? *The FASEB Journal: The Journal of the Federation of American Societies for Experimental Biology*, *20*(7), 858-864. https://doi.org/10.1096/fj.05-4966. com

2. Billman G.E. (2020). Homeostasis: The under appreciated and far too often ignored central organizing principle of physiology. *Frontiers in Physiology*, *11*, Article 200. https://doi.org/10.3389/fphys.2020.00200

3. Brinkman J.E., Dorius B., & Sharma S. (2022). Physiology, body fluids. In *StatPearls*. StatPearls Publishing. https://www.ncbi.nlm.nih.gov/books/NBK482447/

4. Charalampidis C., Youroukou A., Lazaridis G., Baka S., Mpoukovinas I., Karavasilis V., Kioumis I., Pitsiou G., Papaiwannou A., Karavergou A., Tsakiridis K., Katsikogiannis N., Sarika E., Kapanidis K., Sakkas L., Korantzis I., Lampaki S., Zarogoulidis K., & Zarogoulidis P. (2015). Pleura space anatomy. *Journal of thoracic disease*, *7*(1), 27-32. https://doi.org/10.3978/j.issn.2072-1439.2015.01.48

5. Daley M.A., Bramble D.M., & Carrier D.R. (2013). Impact loading and locomotor-respiratory coordination significantly influence breathing dynamics in running humans. *PLOS ONE*, *8*(8). https://doi.org/10.1371/journal.pone.0070752

6. Grover R.F., Weil J.V., & Reeves J.T. (1986). Cardiovascular adaptation to exercise at high altitude. *Exercise & Sport Science Review*, *14*, 269-302. https://pubmed.ncbi.nlm.nih.gov/3525187/

7. Paterson L.Q.P., Amsel R., & Binik Y.M. (2013). Pleasure and pain: The effect of (almost) having an orgasm on genital and nongenital sensitivity. *The Journal of Sexual Medicine*, *10*(6), 1531-1544. https://doi.org/10.1111/jsm.12144

8. Pober J.S., & Sessa W.C. (2015). Inflammation and the blood microvascular system. *Cold Spring Harbor perspectives in biology*, *7*(1), Article a016345. https://doi.org/10.1101/cshperspect.a016345

9. Porter J.L., & Varacallo M. (2022). *Osteoporosis*. In *StatPearls*. StatPearls Publishing. https://www.ncbi.nlm.nih.gov/books/NBK441901/

10. The Editors of Encyclopaedia Britannica (Eds.). (2022, October 7). Vibration. *Encyclopedia Britannica*. https://www.britannica.com/science/vibration

11. Woodard T.L., & Diamond M.P. (2009). Physiologic measures of sexual function in women: A review. *Fertility and Sterility*, *92*(1), 19-34. https://doi.org/10.1016/j.fertnstert.2008.04.041

Chapter 2:

1. Ergen E., Ulkar B. (2007). Chapter 18: Proprioception and coordination. In W.R. Frontera, S. A. Herring, L.J. Micheli,

J.K. Silver, & T.P. Young (Eds.), *Clinical Sports Medicine: Medical Management and Rehabilitation* (pp.237-255). Elsevier. https://doi.org/10.1016/B978-141602443-9.50021-0

2. French A.S., & Torkkeli P.H. (2009). Mechanoreceptors. In *Encyclopedia of Neuroscience* (pp. 689-695). Halifax, Canada: Academic Press. https://doi.org/10.1016/B978-008045046-9.01921-5

3. Merriam-Webster. (n.d.). Fulcrum. In *Merriam-Webster.com dictionary*. Retrieved November 9, 2022, from https://www.merriam-webster.com/dictionary/fulcrum

4. Sun Y., & Tang R. (2019). Tool-use training induces changes of the body scheme in the limb without using tool. *Frontiers in Human Neuroscience, 13,* Article 454. https://doi.org/10.3389/fnhum.2019.00454

Chapter 3:

1. Delgado J., Drinkwater E.J., Banyard H.G., Haff G.G., Nosaka K. (2019). Comparison between back squat, Romanian deadlift, and barbell hip thrust for leg and hip muscle activities during hip extension. *Journal of Strength and Conditioning Research, 33*(10), 2595-2601. https://doi.org/10.1519/JSC.0000000000003290

2. Dunn J., & Grider M.H. (2022). Physiology, Adenosine Triphosphate. In *StatPearls*. StatPearls Publishing. https://www.ncbi.nlm.nih.gov/books/NBK553175/

3. Hussain J., Sundaraj K., Subramaniam I.D., & Lam C.K. (2020). Muscle fatigue in the three heads of triceps brachii during intensity and speed variations of triceps push-down exercise. *Frontiers in Physiology, 11,* Article 112. https://doi.org/10.3389/fphys.2020.00112

4. Ludwig S.A. (2018, July). *Optimization of control parameter for filter algorithms for attitude and heading reference systems* [Conference Paper]. 2018 IEEE Congress on Evolutionary Computation (CEC), Rio de Janeiro, Brazil. https://doi.org/10.1109/CEC.2018.8477725

5. Neto W.K., Soares E.G., Vieria T.L., Aguiar R., Chola T.A., de Lima Sampaio V., & Gama E.F. (2020). Gluteus maximus activation during common strength and hypertrophy exercises: A systematic review. *Journal of Sports Science & Medicine, 19*(1), 195-203. https://www.ncbi.nlm.nih.gov/pmc/articles/PMC7039033/

Chapter 4:

1. Bronstein A.M. (2016). Multisensory integration in balance control. *Handbook of Clinical Neurology, 137*, 57-66. https://doi.org/10.1016/B978-0-444-63437-5.00004-2

2. *Building Bridges: The Basics.* (2017, July 12). MESA. Retrieved November 9, 2022, from https://mesa.ucop.edu/wp-content/uploads/2017/11/2.6-Bridge-Building-Bridges-The-Basics.pdf

3. Eysel-Gosepath K., McCrum C., Epro G., Brüggerman G.-P., & Karamanidis K. (2016). Visual and proprioceptive contribution to postural control of upright stance in unilateral vestibulopathy. *Somatosensory & Motor Research, 33*(2), 72-78. https://doi.org/10.1080/08990220.2016.1178635

4. Han J., Anson J., Waddington G., Adams R., & Liu Y. (2015). The role of ankle proprioception for balance control in relation to sports performance and injury. *Rehabilitation and Improvement of the Postural Function, 2015*, Article 842804. https://doi.org/10.1155/2015/842804

5.   Kennedy P.M., & Inglis J.T. (2002). Distribution and behaviour of glabrous cutaneous receptors in the human foot sole. *The Journal of Physiology*, *538*(Pt 3), 995-1002. https://doi.org/10.1113/jphysiol.2001.013087

6.   Little S. (2022, March 27). *The Arches of the Foot*. Teach Me Anatomy. Retrieved November 9, 2022, from https://teachmeanatomy.info/lower-limb/misc/foot-arches/

7.   Macefield V.G. (2021). The roles of mechanoreceptors in muscle and skin in human proprioception. *Current Opinion in Physiology*, *21*, 48-56. https://doi.org/10.1016/j.cophys.2021.03.003

8.   Manganaro D., & Alsayouri K. (2022). Anatomy, Bony pelvis and lower limb, ankle joint. In *StatPearls*. StatPearls Publishing. https://www.ncbi.nlm.nih.gov/books/NBK545158/

9.   Venkadesan M., Yawar A., Eng C.M., Dias M.A., Singh D.K., Tommasini S.M., Haims A.H., Bandi M.M., & Mandre S. (2020). Stiffness of the human foot and evolution of the transverse arch. *Nature*, (579), 97-100. https://doi.org/10.1038/s41586-020-2053-y

10. Wu C.-C., Chen Y.-J., Hsu C.-S., Wen Y.-T., & Lee Y.-J. (2020). Multiple inertial measurement unit combination and location for center of pressure prediction in gait. *Frontiers in Bioengineering and Biotechnology*, *8*, Article 566474. https://doi.org/10.3389/fbioe.2020.566474

Chapter 5:

1.   Bordoni B., & Varacallo M. (2022). Anatomy, abdomen and pelvis, quadratus lumborum. In *StatPearls*. StatPearls Publishing. https://www.ncbi.nlm.nih.gov/books/NBK535407/

2. Fagard J., Esseily R., Jacquey L., O'Regan K., & Somogyi E. (2018). Fetal origin of sensorimotor behavior. *Frontiers in Neurorobotics, 12*, Article 23. https://doi.org/10.3389/fnbot.2018.00023

3. Gupton M., Munjal A., & Terreberry R.R. (2022). Anatomy, hinge joints. In *StatPearls*. StatPearls Publishing. https://www.ncbi.nlm.nih.gov/books/NBK518967/

4. Hagen D.A., & Valero-Cuevas, F.J. (2017). Similar movements are associated with drastically different muscle contraction velocities. *Journal of Biomechanics, 59*, 90-100. https://doi.org/10.1016/j.jbiomech.2017.05.019

5. Hody S., Croisier J.-L., Bury T., Rogister B., & Leprince P. (2019). Eccentric muscle contractions: Risks and benefits. *Frontiers in Physiology, 10*, Article 536. https://doi.org/10.3389/fphys.2019.00536

6. Jewiss D., Ostman C., & Smart N. (2017). Open versus closed kinetic chain exercises following an anterior cruciate ligament reconstruction: A systematic review and meta-analysis. *Journal of Sports Medicine, 2017*, Article 4721548. https://doi.org/10.1155/2017/4721548

7. Makin T.R., Diedrichsen J., & Krakauer J.W. (2020). Reorganization in adult primate sensorimotor cortex: Does it really happen? In Poeppel D., Mangun G.R., & Gazzaniga M.S. (Eds.), *The Cognitive Neurosciences* (6th ed.). The MIT Press. https://doi.org/10.7551/mitpress/11442.003.0057

8. Pitch, yaw, and roll. (2022, May 3). In *Wikipedia*. https://simple.wikipedia.org/wiki/Pitch,_yaw,_and_roll

9. Ristroph L., Ristroph G., Morozova S., & Bergou A. (2013). Active and passive stabilization of body pitch in insect flight. *Journal of the Royal Society Interface, 10*(85). https://doi.org/10.1098/rsif.2013.0237

10. Vaienti E., Scita G., Ceccarelli F., & Pogliacomi F. (2017). Understanding the human knee and its relationship to total knee replacement. *Acta Biomedica: Atenei Parmensis*, *88*(S2): 6-16. https://www.ncbi.nlm.nih.gov/pmc/articles/PMC6178997/

11. Vimal V.P., Lackner J.R., & DiZio P. (2018). Learning dynamic control of body yaw orientation. *Experimental Brain Research*, *236*(5), 1321-1330. https://doi.org/10.1007/s00221-018-5216-4

Chapter 6:

1. Barnish M.S., & Barnish J. (2016, January 13). High-heeled shoes and musculoskeletal injuries: A narrative systematic review. *BMJ Open*, *6*(1). https://doi.org/10.1136/bmjopen-2015-010053

2. Behm D.G., Peach A., Maddigan M., Aboodarba S.J., DiSanto M.C., Button D.C., & Maffiuletti N.A. (2013, October). Massage and stretching reduce spinal reflex excitability without affecting twitch contractile properties. *Journal of Electromyography and Kinesiology*, *23*(5), 1215-1221. https://doi.org/10.1016/j.jelekin.2013.05.002

3. Borchgrevink G.E., Viset A.T., Witsø E., Schei B., & Foss O.A. (2016, December). Does the use of high-heeled shoes lead to fore-foot pathology? A controlled cohort study comprising 197 women. *Foot and Ankle Surgery*, *22*(4), 239-243. https://doi.org/10.1016/j.fas.2015.10.004

4. Bordoni B., Sugumar K., & Varacallo M. (2022, September 4). Muscle cramps. In *StatPearls*. StatPearls Publishing. https://www.ncbi.nlm.nih.gov/books/NBK499895/

5. Bridge Masters. (2017, March 12). How it works: Engineering bridges to handle stress. https://bridgemastersinc.com/engineering-bridges-handle-stress/

6. Elftman H. (1969, Spring). Dynamic structure of the human foot. *Artificial Limbs*, *13*(1), 49-58. http://www.oandplibrary.org/al/1969_01_049.asp

7. Galbusera F., & Bassani T. (2019). The spine: A strong, stable, and flexible structure with biomimetics potential. *Biomimetics*, *4*(3), 60. https://doi.org/10.3390/biomimetics4030060

8. Giuriato G., Pedrinolla A., Schena F., & Venturelli M. (2018, August). Muscle cramps: A comparison of the two-leading hypothesis. *Journal of Electromyography and Kinesiology*, *41*, 89-95. https://doi.org/10.1016/j.jelekin.2018.05.006

9. Guissard N., & Duchateau J. (2006, October). Neural aspects of muscle stretching. *Exercise and Sport Sciences Reviews*, *34*(4), 154-158. https://doi.org/10.1249/01.jes.0000240023.30373.eb

10. Gwani A.S., Asari M.A., & Ismail Z.I.M. (2017). How the three arches of the foot intercorrelate. *Folia Morphologica*, *76*(4), 682-688. https://pubmed.ncbi.nlm.nih.gov/28553850/

11. Johns, T. (2010, January 7). *What is a keystone?* ASU- Ask A Biologist. https://askabiologist.asu.edu/what-keystone

12. Kaur K., & Sinha A.G.K. (2020, October 1). Effectiveness of massage on flexibility of hamstring muscle and agility of female players: An experimental randomized controlled trial. *Journal of Bodywork and Movement Therapies*, *24*(4), 519-526. https://doi.org/10.1016/j.jbmt.2020.06.029

13. Madhok S.S., & Shabbir N. (2022, September 12). Hypotonia. In *StatPearls*. StatPearls Publishing. https://pubmed.ncbi.nlm.nih.gov/32965880/

14. Medline Plus. (2020, December 3). *Your baby in the birth canal*. https://medlineplus.gov/ency/article/002060.htm

15. Merriam-Webster. (n.d.). Stability. In *Merriam-Webster.com dictionary*. Retrieved November 18, 2022, from https://www.merriam-webster.com/dictionary/stability

16. Miller T.M., & Layer R.B. (2005, October). Muscle cramps. *Muscle & Nerve, 32*(4), 431-442. https://doi.org/10.1002/mus.20341

17. Nichols T.R., Huyghues-Despointes C.M.J.I. (2009). Muscular stiffness. In M.D. Binder, N. Hirokawa, U. Windhorst (Eds.), *Encyclopedia of Neuroscience* (pp.2515-2519). Springer, Berlin, Heidelberg. https://doi.org/10.1007/978-3-540-29678-2_3687

18. Pabón M.A.M., & Naqvi U. (2022, May 29). Achilles tendonitis. In *StatPearls*. StatPearls Publishing. https://www.ncbi.nlm.nih.gov/books/NBK538149/

19. Pate R., Oria M., & Pillsbury L. (Eds.). (2012, December 10). Heath-related fitness measures for youth: Flexibility. In *Fitness Measures and Health Outcomes in Youth*. National Academies Press. https://www.ncbi.nlm.nih.gov/books/NBK241323/

20. Roberts T.J. (2016, January). Contribution of elastic tissues to the mechanics and energetics of muscle function during movement. *Journal of Experimental Biology, 219*(Pt. 2), 266-275. https://doi.org/https://pubmed.ncbi.nlm.nih.gov/26792339/

21. Samim M., Moukaddam H.A., Smitaman E. (2016, August). Imaging of Mueller-Weiss syndrome: A review of clinical presentations and imaging spectrum. *American Journal of Roentgenology, 207*, 8-18. https://doi.org/10.2214/AJR.15.15843

22. Saunders F.R., Gregory J.S., Pavlova A.V., Muthuri S.G., Hardy R.J., Martin K.R., Barr R.J., Adams J.E., Kuh D., Aspden R.M., Cooper R., & Ireland A. (2020, March 12). Motor development in infancy and spine shape in early old age: Findings from a British birth cohort study. *Journal of Orthopaedic Research, 38*(12), 2740-2748. https://doi.org/10.1002/jor.24656

23. Swash M., Czesnik D., & de Carvalho M. (2019, February). Muscular cramp: Causes and management. *European Journal of Neurology, 26*(2), 214-221. https://doi.org/10.1111/ene.13799

24. Thesaurus.com. (n.d.). Stiff. In *Thesaurus.com thesaurus*. Retrieved October 27, 2022, from https://www.thesaurus.com/browse/stiff

25. Vasavada A., Ward S.R., Delp S., & Lieber R.L. (2010). Architectural design and function of human back muscles. In *Herkowitz_Chapter 3*. https://nmbl.stanford.edu/publications/pdf/Vasavada2010.pdf

26. Wiedemeijer M.M., & Otten E. (2018, March). Effects of high heeled shoes on gait. A review. *Gait & Posture, 61*, 423-430. https://doi.org/10.1016/j.gaitpost.2018.01.036

27. Wirth K., Hartmann H., Mickel C., Szilvas E., Keiner M., & Sander A. (2017, March). Core stability in athletes: A critical analysis of current guidelines. *Sports Medicine, 47*(3), 401-414. https://doi.org/10.1007/s40279-016-0597-7

Appendix:

1. Let's Talk Science. (2020, March 09). *Simple Machines - Levers*. https://letstalkscience.ca/educational-resources/backgrounders/simple-machines-levers

2. Science Learning Hub. (2007, June 21). *What levers does your body use?* Curious Minds. https://www.sciencelearn. org.nz/resources/1924-what-levers-does-your-body-use

3. Taylor, T. (2017, October 27). *1ˢᵗ Class Lever*. Innerbody. https://www.innerbody.com/image_musc04/musc73.html

www.ingramcontent.com/pod-product-compliance
Lightning Source LLC
Chambersburg PA
CBHW070112030426
42335CB00016B/2123